A LIFE
Yet to Live

A LIFE
Yet to Live

Finding Health, Vitality, and Joy **after 60**

RON KASTNER

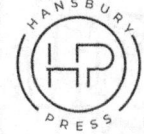

Published in the USA by
Hansbury Press
www.RonKastner.com

Copyright © 2023 Ron Kastner
All rights reserved under International and Pan-American Copyright Conventions.

Publisher's Note:
Without limiting the rights under copyright reserved above, no part of this publication may be reproduced, stored or introduced into a retrieval system or transmitted, in any form, or by any means (electronic, photocopying, recording, or otherwise), without the prior written permission of both the copyright owner and the above publisher of this book.

For information about permission to reproduce selections from this book:
info@RonKastner.com
Please put Permissions in the subject line.

Names: Kastner, Ron, 1950– author.
Title: A life yet to live : finding health, vitality, and joy after 60 / Ron Kastner.
Description: [New York, New York] : Hansbury Press, [2023] | Includes bibliographical references and index.
Identifiers: ISBN: 979-8-218-25047-8 (paperbound) | 979-8-218-25048-5 (eBook) | LCCN: 2023914646
Subjects: LCSH: Longevity. | Aging. | Vitality. | Health. | Exercise. | Physical fitness. | Well-being—Age factors. | Aging—Nutritional aspects. | Older people—Health and hygiene. | Older people—Life skills guides. | LCGFT: Self-help publications. | BISAC: HEALTH & FITNESS / Longevity. | HEALTH & FITNESS / Exercise / General. | SELF-HELP / Aging.
Classification: LCC: RA776.75 | DDC: 612.6/8—dc23

To Jess and Lollie,
To Lollie and Jess,
Not first and second
Or second and first,
But the twin stars
In whose orbits I have come to spin.

This is what I leave you,
A letter long in the making.
May you live your lives
By your own flesh and blood,
And your own inner light.

CONTENTS

PART I	FIRST STEPS	1
	A Life Yet to Live: *The Gift of Mortality*	
CHAPTER 1	A Train Ride to New Jersey	11
CHAPTER 2	Detox and a Lesson in Nutrition	21
CHAPTER 3	Four Doctors	37
CHAPTER 4	Born to Move	53
CHAPTER 5	Profound Change Begins	69
CHAPTER 6	The World Within	81
CHAPTER 7	Serendipity: *Letting Life Guide Me*	89
CHAPTER 8	Healing a Family Disaster	97
CHAPTER 9	The Great Guide	105
PART II	MY LIFE PRACTICE	111
	A New Definition of Health	
CHAPTER 10	Power and Its Cousins: *Energy, Strength, Endurance, and Vitality*	127
CHAPTER 11	Fuel: *What Keeps Us Operating*	137
CHAPTER 12	To Live Is to Move	165
CHAPTER 13	Balance, Alignment, and Posture	181
CHAPTER 14	Recovery, Repair, and Renewal	193

CHAPTER 15   Clarity, Grace, Wisdom, and Serenity. 213

CHAPTER 16   Metrics, Diagnosis, and Support 225

PART III   FRUITS OF THE JOURNEY. .237

CHAPTER 17   Parenting: *A Universal Journey* 239

CHAPTER 18   Modern Life: *Friend or Foe?* 249

CHAPTER 19   Vanity: *Attempts to Look Young* 263

CHAPTER 20   Genes: *The Role They Play* 269

CHAPTER 21   When Bad Stuff Happens:
             Three Lessons in Healing. 277

CONCLUSION   Loving Life: *The Endless Journey* 301

ENDNOTES 305

RESOURCES 308

SELECTED BIBLIOGRAPHY. 320

ACKNOWLEDGMENTS 333

ABOUT THE AUTHOR. 334

INDEX 336

PART I

First Steps

A Life Yet to Live
The Gift of Mortality

"Through the whole of life, one must continue to learn to live."
—SENECA

"The privilege of a lifetime is being who you are."
—JOSEPH CAMPBELL

What does the rest of my life have in store for me?

This question marked where I started the journey I've been on for about fifteen years. As I was approaching age sixty, I had what I call a "mortality moment"—a profound realization that I was entering later life—the third act of life—and that this period would be my last on this planet. Once I allowed that moment to sink in and followed where it led me, everything I believed about life itself changed. The moment turned into one of clarity and depth, the likes of which I had rarely experienced.

Heading toward or becoming sixty seems to be a potentially pivotal age in life. Each of us experiences it differently, but I would venture a hunch that turning sixty includes contemplating our lives as well as wondering what the future holds, along with the full range of emotions we feel when contemplating our existence. In her book *The Top Five Regrets of the Dying*, palliative care nurse Bronnie Ware states that the most common regret is the wish to have "lived the life they wanted to instead of living as others expected them to." She writes about the heartbreaking story of a woman telling her this deep regret toward the end of her life, with no time left to change. Perhaps at sixty, there is still enough time left to change and discover the lives we want or are meant to lead? For me, this journey began at age fifty-eight.

All at once, my priorities became clear and unavoidable: a combination of loving my two then very young daughters, establishing a practice for health and longevity, and addressing the longings inside me for a genuine, wholehearted life. Despite my successful career and the deeply satisfying start of my family, I realized what had eluded me. Genuineness and wholeheartedness were missing.

In the years since that mortality moment, I've lived on a bumpy and often conflicting path navigating the intertwined worlds of parenting, becoming healthy, and knowing my inner spirit. At age seventy-three, I am healthier, stronger, more energetic, more grounded, a better parent, and more at home in my own flesh and blood than I've ever been. The limits I had lived with were largely internal. Suddenly, I was given a great gift: the ability to experience life from the inside out and occupy my body as the visceral being I am.

Today, I am grateful every day for the preciousness of being alive, a 24/7 process I had only glimpsed before. Yet this largely unseen and unappreciated inner spirit has been alive inside me all along. A big part of my journey called for removing the obstacles that kept me from feeling its power, a process that continues every day.

In conversations with others, I realize we all have these mortality moments at different ages and stages. Some of us hear them, and some try to shut them out to continue life as usual. But that comes at our peril or at least at our loss. Our bodies keep sending us deep messages to heed. For me, it said, "Make the most of the time you have left." By following that message, the quality of my health and inner life has changed profoundly.

Whatever that message is to each of us, it comes from a place inside that's the essence of *who we are*. Call it soul, conscience, or spirit; it is our true center that means us only good, even if it feels fearful at first.

THE MIRACLE OF HEALTH AND LIFE

The ultimate source of health and longevity comes not from a doctor, or a supplement, or exercise, or a healthy diet. While these can be useful tools, health *itself* is the miraculous system living within us, a system of myriad complexity and wonder.

We are all born with this gift from the universe. What happens in our bodies is an infinite cascade of miracles. Yet we mostly take them for granted until they don't function well. I now devote my days to appreciating both life and health. I know the ultimate source of health goes back to the beginnings of time, to the source of existence. Living in harmony with that source serves me today in the best way possible—the way the universe created us.

When I first experienced my mortality moment, my priority became *having time*—especially having time to be a good father to my two young daughters. This translated not only into spending more hours together but extending my physical health, energy, and well-being for as long as possible. As a father who had children in his fifties, I wanted *longevity with highly functional health*, so I consumed as much information as I could on how to prolong my vitality. Through trial and error, hunch and inspiration, I've come up with practices that involve all aspects of life that have worked wonders for me on many fronts. And contrary to what many would have us believe, I've found that my biological health is intertwined with my emotional, mental, and spiritual life.

At first, I thought that physical health was *only* a matter of exercise and diet, the two mainstays of a preventive health practice. Naturally, they provide a good place to start. But as my body grew stronger and began to heal, I realized that body and mind are not separate entities. Their integration and long evolutionary history contribute to who I am today. A big part of me—the unconscious part that controls my health—operates on a rhythm and cadence that's aligned with the beating heart of the universe. The body's autonomic system is responsible for the myriad miraculous processes that maintain or improve health. Thus, achieving good preventive health aims at enhancing this system.

Many of the integrated practices I follow are rooted in ancient traditions such as yoga and natural foods; some are more recent such as psychotherapy and high-intensity interval training (HIIT). But all are based on a fundamental reconnection with the wonder of how body, mind, and spirit work *and* the awe of health itself. Once I had experienced this primal connection to my visceral body and all it's capable of—in movement, thought, emotion, and spirit—a new world opened.

MODERN MEDICINE AND HEALTH

Modern medicine has much to offer in the way of intervening and fixing what's wrong with us symptomatically. Targeted antibiotics and effective surgery are two of its biggest triumphs. But it has surprisingly little to offer for curing the underlying conditions that plague our later years and preventing those conditions from appearing in the first place. Much of that quest relates to one's lifestyle or lifestyle *changes*. And while traditional doctors are slowly coming around to emphasizing how diet, movement, and lifestyle affect health, they still have a long way to go.

Luckily, a host of integrative doctors and researchers as well as networks of people sharing their experiences are making our health stories more complete. Yet, getting people to take these integrative messages to heart is still an uphill battle. Why the hesitation? Because a journey to optimum health starts from inside, fostering changes in how we appreciate ourselves and deem if we're worth the effort. This is trickier territory than knowing what foods to eat or how much to exercise. Even integrative practitioners have conflicting or self-promoting advice at times, making the questions of which path to follow and who to trust even more complicated.

For instance, we simply don't yet know enough about how our bodies integrate with mind, spirit, and belief. Yet evidence indicates this connection is vast. Nor do we appreciate how much harm poor diet and lack of movement have done to our health. I've found that a blended approach, drawing from old and new, Eastern and Western, serves me best—along with knowing that every part of me affects every other part. It begs the question, "How can we categorize the vastness of health and quality of life by tests and metrics in a doctor's office?"

FUNDAMENTALS OF SELF-HEALTH

I'm not a scientist nor a doctor nor an expert. I simply want to stick around a long time to experience life fully. In addition to readily available information and sources, I turn to my own growing instinctual feel for health. I have worked hard at it, tried new things, and come to know myself better in the process. The ideas in this book reflect how I've learned to rely on my judgment and uncover the inner power required to navigate vast amounts of information.

The fundamentals I have learned in my health journey have changed the way I spend my time. The center of the whole effort is dictated by my own self-value: what I want out of life, what matters to me, what makes me tick. In turn, being the healthiest me is the best way to interact with those I love and the world around me.

Once I experienced healthiness on the inside as the multifaceted gift it is, all my practices became aimed at supporting wholeness in my life for years to come.

HOW I DEFINE HEALTH

Health has as many definitions as the people who use it. To me, health is the system of equilibrium, energy, and growth the universe has given me. Healing is part of the same system that drives everything in the living world. But health is also a state that allows me to experience my truest nature and live as genuinely and wholeheartedly as possible. The more I focus on staying healthy in a full sense and practice self-health by caring for my whole being, the more I affirm how my emotional and spiritual life are intricately tied to my physical body. Like an iceberg, 90 percent of one's awareness is hidden. Because emotions, dreams, biochemistry, and belief mix mostly under the surface, I do my best to bring this extended form of self-health to the surface.

Self-health is ultimately self-love and self-worth, both of which I've discovered along the way. What helped me change a previously less-than-loving attitude toward myself is my increasingly strong goal of being healthy in a universal sense. The more I practice self-love and self-worth, the stronger this sense of universal health becomes.

NEW LIFE PATH

My new path differs greatly from my old one. It's largely inner driven and less obviously ambitious. It has more clarity, more simple joy, and fewer robotic social elements. My path is less confusing and conflicted, more grounded with added space and richness. My journey is especially more genuine and wholehearted, quieter and more comfortably solitary. Today, I am less concerned with the *circumstances* of life than with life itself. Ego and wealth pale in importance. Rather, I am constantly curious, filled with awe for the world both outside and inside me.

I am less afraid of new ideas or emotions or memories or people than I used to be. I also realize how most stress and anger are caused by emotional dynamics *inside* me. Being more aware, I can tolerate these and other unpleasant emotions to uncover their dynamics, loosening their grip on me.

I have gained a healthy respect, a sixth sense for what's working and what isn't. I find clarity and enjoyment in much of daily living, despite regular doubts and wobbles that need sorting through. Along the way, I've become fit, thin, and strong. Most important, I have evolved a strategy for my remaining years, one that keeps me moving and growing. I have an ever-bigger toolbox for when I get stuck or sick. And I work toward my priorities most days. Even the "off" recovery days serve their vital purpose.

Being forced to experience my mortality moment is a gift for which I will forever feel grateful. This encounter taught me to see what I want from the rest of my life—front row center.

A LIFE YET TO LIVE

I'm proposing an entirely new chapter of existence at this late stage of life. That's not new. Traditions in many cultures highly value the profound uniqueness of life past age sixty. The Hindus have Sannyasa, the period of later life of renunciation and a turn toward spirit. The Japanese have ikigai, finding one's true purpose in life, which is a mainstay of much of its longer-lived culture. Many traditions of elderhood, both ancient and modern, revere the singular wisdom provided by the vast experience of older people. Many of these qualities can't be learned; they can only be acquired by having experienced life.

Our modern world has so many diversions from these practices—including seeking youth—that we have lost much of our ability to value our later years. In my case, when I stopped chasing youth and squarely faced my mortality, youthful spirit and energy found *me*.

1

A Train Ride to New Jersey

"To pay attention, this is our endless and proper work."
—MARY OLIVER

"Follow your passion."
—JOSEPH CAMPBELL

My journey started on a train ride from New York to New Jersey on an icy cold winter's day in late 2007. This train ride came to define my life so momentously that I will refer to it often in this manuscript. I'd taken this route many times, having grown up in Newark and been pulled to nearby New York City. That vast mecca of energy that felt like Oz when I was young became the place I spent most of my adult life. "Making it there," as the Frank Sinatra song says, became my mission for years.

On this midwinter day with bright blue skies, brilliant sunshine, a bone-chilling temperature, and a brisk Artic-like wind, I had to keep moving to avoid being cold. I was on my way to a business meeting in Secaucus, New Jersey, ushering in the beginning of what became a long, painful process of selling the printing company I'd started with a team of co-employees eighteen years earlier. Capital Printing Systems, Inc. had provided me with a platform for personal growth, change, and wealth I had never expected. We had built it into a profitable enterprise, but it was experiencing trouble due to the impending US financial crisis.

Financial printing is a highly specialized business serving Wall Street customers by producing prospectuses and other documents for complicated financial transactions. The documents themselves were books—often several hundred pages of legal wording. Called "disclosures" by the lawyers and Securities and Exchange Commission (SEC) who oversaw the process, these printed materials described transactions and their risk factors.

Our staff would take all the mess of files, charts, notes, and scribbles that described the deal in question (provided by lawyers, bankers, and accountants) and assemble them into a professionally typeset and readable format. Over weeks or months, we revised the documents and circulated them for approval through countless cycles before the actual printing took place. Our work had to be done quickly, precisely, and accurately, which required being open twenty-four hours a day and six or seven days a week. Although running this business was challenging, doing it well meant a lot of money could be made.

I started this printing company when I was forty years old after a ten-year stint as a salesman with a similar firm. My business had not only made me wealthy beyond my wildest blue-collar dreams; it enabled me to stretch the definition of "me" to include "successful entrepreneur, boss, and businessman." Indirectly, it also led to my co-career as an award-winning New York and London theater and film producer.

At one point I was literally a highflier. With others, I was even profiled in a Newsweek article titled "NYLON" (as in New York and London). We were people who called both cities home, flying back and forth, sometimes via Concorde, for both work and pleasure.

COMPANY STARTED TO CRUMBLE

That day on the commuter train to New Jersey, the world I'd built for myself and my family had started to crumble. The extent to which the company's success had come to underpin my future was apparent in the anxiety I felt after its sudden decline in the summer of 2007. That's when our thriving pipeline of deals suddenly slowed down, marking the rumblings of what became the full-blown financial crisis of 2008. Capital Printing Systems, Inc. was like the canary in the coal mine with early tremors felt in Wall Street and London, where we had a second office.

Yet the trepidation I felt was not only about supporting my family and our tasteful yet affluent lifestyle. In addition to homes in New York and London, we enjoyed summer getaways, exotic vacations, and extravagant entertaining. While not "private jet" wealthy, I had enough assets to make huge purchases without a second thought. The image of how I moved through the world as a "success" was my mirror. Status and money had given me confidence and opened doors I thought I never could access. But that year, the status (or armor) I used to value myself was in danger.

This harbinger trip to New Jersey marked the first of many negotiation meetings as I struggled to sell the company before its demise. An undercurrent of sheer terror set in over the months as I let go of this golden goose with sales of $70 million a year.

Still, life was about to hand me a gift amid the chaos—one that, over time, became far more important than the crisis itself. I had experienced a professional crisis before in 1990 when the financial printing firm I worked for was in trouble and sold off its divisions, one of which I purchased and formed Capital. Yet the gift about to drop into my lap on this train ride was different, letting loose something deep inside that became more important than wealth, success, or status. In fact, a light shined on the opposite. I thank the forces of the universe—and what I call the unfathomable insights of my inner and outer worlds—for bringing me to that point. In retrospect, I was delivered such an extraordinary confluence of factors that, on some cosmic level, the experience must have been planned.

AN OWNER'S MANUAL ON STAYING YOUNG

After making my way to Penn Station by subway that day, I picked up a book at Borders bookstore to pass the time. It was titled *You, Staying Young: The Owner's Manual for Extending Your Warranty* and written by two doctors, Michael Roizen and Mehmet Oz. (This happened when Dr. Oz was still a practicing surgeon and before he became a media name and politician.) The book discussed how we age and what we can do to extend our lives.

Instinctively, I picked up the book and leafed through it. I guess I was so ready to immerse myself in this subject that everything I read struck a chord—about how the body works, why different parts and organs show signs of age, and what can be done to prevent them from wearing out. Most important, I read that the kind of weak and resigned old age I had witnessed didn't need to be a foregone conclusion for everyone, including me. How exciting!

The train made its way out of Manhattan, rumbling through the tunnels under the Hudson River into the wide-open blue skies of the Meadowlands in New Jersey. The subject of this book had already triggered a flood of associations, emotions, memories, and thoughts that came at me like a faster version of the train I rode.

I can't do justice to describing the fifteen-minute ride to Secaucus. My body tingled all over, no doubt fueled by the pressure I felt in selling the company. This book represented a brighter future than the worry-laden one I was facing. No doubt I was also affected by the geography of the trip itself—moving toward my childhood home.

But as events have played out, this train ride represented more than all that. I call it the thunderbolt of a wake-up call that came simultaneously from inside and outside. It fueled a chain reaction setting everything in motion as if a long-dormant machine suddenly sprang into action. A deep visceral chord had been awakened in my gut. Here's what I remember as best as I can express it.

TRIGGERED MEMORIES OF MY YOUTH

The two main poles of my geographical life had been New Jersey and New York City. The train ride triggered memories of my youth in Newark and of making this journey countless times before, as if, in heading that direction, I was revisiting my early life. Farther down this same track was the Weequahic section of Newark where I grew up, the cemeteries in Iselin where my parents and grandparents are buried, and the buildings in New Brunswick where I went to college at Rutgers.

While I have fond memories of those times, one overwhelming emotion sat on top of them all and has for my entire life—loss, the hole left in my life when my father died. The emotion from his passing and its aftermath took over my life. At the time, he was forty-seven years old, and I was seven. He died of pancreatic cancer, its presence and treatment monopolizing his last few years. This train ride, the book in my hands, my current circumstances, and a vast array of forces at work combined to produce a wondrous insight within me at that moment.

I sat on the train as it rolled toward Secaucus through the great wetland and former garbage dump. Memories, perceptions, and emotions swirled inside me as I had never felt them before. I sensed my father's absence deep inside of me so much, I wished he were present to comfort and guide me through my current troubles.

At the exact time, another insight about my life made a parallel entrance, one that years of therapy and remembering had never moved me as much. I became crystal clear that I felt my loss so deeply because I had two young children of my own. I felt a giant responsibility to them. Even if nothing medically catastrophic happened to me, as an older father, I'd be sentencing my daughters to a fate like mine *simply by going through the slow decline in ability and health known as aging.* As had happened to me, they would miss having a father in the prime of life, unable to give them everything they deserved in the way of love, participation, energy, and support. I felt a fear of what had happened to me returning full circle, and I was feeling that fear for *them.*

This was not about financial support or being the best dad I could be. It was about being *present, alive, and fully functional for them.* The doctors' book that had catalyzed this whole subject seemed to hold the answer, offering a way to avoid repeating what had happened to me, feeling stuck in the past with no way out. How could I let that same fate befall my children?

What answers? For me, information in the Roizen and Oz book opened possibilities of slowing the aging process. I could hope to maintain my health, vitality, strength, and flexibility, and maybe buy extra time on this earth. I sensed a resurgence of hope. Yes, I could do something to soften what had seemed like an inescapable fate. I wouldn't be dodging death exactly but ensuring the biggest priority was to stay vital long enough to be an involved and present dad to my daughters.

MOMENTS OF POWERFUL INSIGHT

The Buddhists say that enlightenment (or windows of insight that allow people to receive inspiration from a mysterious source deep within) allows one to experience all three tenses—past, present, and future, as well as one's inner and outer life—in one seamless experience of the here and now. Although I can't explain or re-create what happened to me on the train ride, I can say it was all powerful. The encounter emerged as a unity of cause, effect, and future action, an "aha" moment. My eyes opened, and I "got it."

Although I'm not a Buddhist, I've learned a great deal more about Buddhism since then. These moments of insight are not about cause and effect, subject and object. Rather, they are the living embodiment of the miraculous power of synthesizing all aspects of experience, thought, and feeling in which our souls can participate. We see many versions of these insights in religion, art, and life. The world suddenly makes sense in a different way and so we see it differently. We only have to allow ourselves to accept such insight without being bound by limitations. "Be who you truly are, and all things will become clear." "Coming to terms with the world inside us shapes our world outside."

The moment flashed by quickly. I became so absorbed in the memories, the book's messages, and my life at that point that I barely noticed the train had pulled into the Secaucus station. I still had years of putting on my business face to get through these meetings, but I chose to focus more on thinking about my daughters, living a healthy life, and pursuing the promise of longevity.

MY DECLINE NOT INEVITABLE

On the way back to Manhattan, I finished reading the Roizen and Oz book and later picked up a similar recommended book called *Younger Next Year* by Chris Crowley and Dr. Henry Lodge. I devoured it as well. The authors explained that the seemingly inevitable decline of aging is not a given, provided we follow lifestyle changes that involve exercise, diet, and positive mental outlook. The text discussed what our bodies were made for and how different levels of aerobic exercise (in particular, the necessary movement of our prehistoric ancestors) can keep us at highly functional levels well into our seventies, eighties, and nineties.

And something else happened on that train ride, something I was only fuzzily aware of and couldn't tease apart from everything else. This realization arrived at a cost to my previous notion of personal security based on success and superiority. And my mortality was being addressed in a way it never had been before.

Yes, I realized I was fearful of aging, dying, infirmity, disease, and not being able to enjoy a fully functioning body, mind, and soul. As a wealthy friend bluntly stated, "I would give it all up for more time and better health." My fear also centered on not being present and active for my children as they grew up. However, I admit much of my apprehension related to my deep sense of *wanting to do more* with my remaining years. I felt as if part of me hadn't yet lived. I yearned to step into a new life, shouting, "What do you mean it's almost over? I haven't even started yet!"

This wake-up call told me I still wanted to do much—not only for my family but for *me*—and I needed time, health, and energy for that. *Is there more left in me to know and experience? Is there a part of me that hasn't yet expressed itself or been realized?* I admitted to feeling a gnawing emptiness when I asked these questions.

Luckily, the path I'd been shown on this momentous train ride eventually held answers to these questions. Health, parenting, longevity, and self-experience were not separate provinces to be explored in cookie-cutter fashion. All are wondrous, intertwined aspects of being alive, guided by the miraculous wonder of *who I am* and *how I got here*.

Thus, a new and profoundly different era began for me. And these years have proven to be a wellspring of health, vitality, and joy in magnitudes I never expected.

2

Detox and a Lesson in Nutrition

"When you get to the root cause or causes, so many often-related symptoms go away without having to be addressed individually."
—DR. MARK HYMAN

After my experience on the train ride to Secaucus, I continued reading and learning as much as I could. But day-to-day life and supporting my family preempted any substantial health practices other than continuing some yoga, going to the gym occasionally, and walking as much as I could. My diet didn't change, nor did my drinking, for at least another year.

Selling my company was harder and more stressful than anything I had ever done. And after it was all over, I tried to restore my previous successes in both business and theater. I started working on three new businesses while I also produced a few plays in London's West End. On many levels, I felt like a failure for what had happened with the printing company. It wasn't just about money (we had enough to live well). I needed the admiration that came with success and wealth, so I drove myself hard to recapture what I had lost. In the end, one of the businesses worked well and the others dried up. Typically, the plays had mixed results.

My first important health effort was a three-week detox

recommended by a good friend and yoga instructor of more than two decades, Nikki Costello. She pointed me toward the book *Clean* by Dr. Alejandro Junger.

The theory presented in *Clean* struck a chord with me—that is, we need to allow our bodies time to heal by reducing our food intake and eliminating possible inflammatory toxins in our diet. I had never been exposed to anything like this other than reading about the calorie restriction studies and their beneficial effects on longevity. Junger's theories were the product of his own burnout as a critical care cardiologist. Burnout forced him to turn to the preventive side of health to help people *before* they got to the emergency room.

This was my first venture into what I call "deep health," addressing its underground dynamics. People rarely have the guts to experience both the absence of daily comfort as well as the unconventionality that goes with radical experimentation with cleanses. When I tried a cleanse, though, it changed most of my beliefs about what causes disease *and* contributed to the miraculous benefits of practicing self-care.

A ROBUST IMMUNE SYSTEM

The author of *Clean* explains why and how many types of food might stress our immune system—the living, breathing center of our bodies' defense and repair processes. Dr. Junger writes that a healthy immune system is continuously active, balanced, and selective. It's constantly on the alert for toxins, including foreign invaders such as parasites or viruses, as well as existing cells that are no longer useful or downright harmful. Those vary from irritants and allergens to cells that are malformed, dead, or past their "use-by" date. Included is a whole range of things our bodies don't need or are directly disease causing—including cancer cells, plaque cells, and parasites. These badly made or harmful cells, along with waste products and unwelcome guests, require removal that won't interfere with healthy tissue. The healthier the immune system is, the more robust, selective, and discriminating it can be when finding and disposing of potentially harmful cells. The cells are either invaders or have outlived their usefulness and can cause problems. The sooner they are eliminated, the better.

If we overload our vital immune system by not giving it enough time or energy to do its job or by ingesting too many foods requiring its attention, we compromise its effectiveness. It weakens and loses its ability to discriminate between friend and foe.

Dr. Junger's three-week cleanse program calls for eliminating any possible immune response–triggering foods from our diet. In theory, once our immune system isn't bombarded with toxins, its natural strength returns. In practice, it was time for my immune system to begin the process of deep cleaning.

THE ABCS OF IMMUNITY

The immune system is made up of the infinitely complex processes of intra- and intercellular metabolism as well as many types of white blood and lymph cells that are on constant patrol. They surround or ingest toxic elements, including cellular waste and dead or dysfunctional cells, thereby neutralizing them. They then float through the bloodstream to be eliminated by either the liver or kidneys. All this happens trillions of times a day. I am in awe of this biochemically intricate process that's working every second, yet people are largely unaware of it and rarely see or feel it in action.

Previously, I thought my immune system went into gear only

when faced with an illness, a virus or bacteria, or an injury. Yet, given enough time and energy to perform its job, the immune system accomplishes amazing feats of housekeeping. It keeps me humming and healthy at all times. Before long, I realized that keeping my immune system at peak levels would enhance my longevity goals.

According to Dr. Junger in *Clean* (and a newer version called *Clean Gut*), our modern lifestyles, environment, and diet have introduced a new array of toxins to worry about—in addition to those that have been around a few hundred years. The result? A flood of internal damage that our bodies don't have the time or resources to clean up. Without realizing it, most of us overwhelm our bodies with toxins. But the foods eliminated during the *Clean* program have been scientifically shown to trigger reactions and can needlessly overtax our immune systems.

In an overwhelmed system, rather than cleaning as we go, our immune function tends to stay on red alert like an ambulance or medical crew that never rests. It then starts doing triage instead of treatment and can make poor decisions. Immune system malfunctions can allow toxicity to gain a toehold and gradually become a bigger threat than ever. Heart disease, diabetes, and a host of other chronic disorders owe their mild beginnings to low immune function.

An immune system that is less efficient and discriminating creates our greatest risk for developing chronic disease. In extreme cases, an overworked immune system can't discriminate between healthy and unhealthy tissue and begins to attack cells of its own body if they resemble toxins it has encountered in the past. This "autoimmune" aspect is another indicator of compromised immunity, becoming the basis for many diseases such as multiple sclerosis, rheumatoid arthritis, and Crohn's disease, to name a few.

THREE WEEKS OF DETOXING

The three weeks it takes to effectively do the *Clean* detox can be daunting for modern lifestyles. I certainly found this to be true. The prescribed detox involves restrictions on food and dramatically changes one's eating habits. This means no alcohol, caffeine, sugar, dairy, wheat (or anything else with gluten), and eliminating certain fruits and vegetables. Included is only fresh food, preferably organic or as "natural" as possible—nothing processed. As author Michael Pollan writes in *Food Rules*, "If it comes from a plant, eat it; if it was made in a plant, don't."[1] In short, if it comes in a box, it's probably not food.

Each of us reacts differently to various types of food. Beyond preferences, we experience visceral reactions caused by our natural genetic, emotional, or physical makeup. One size does not fit all.

Fueled by my own informed practices and experimentation, I've found a customized approach most effective. The same goes once my detox ends. As I reintroduce other kinds of food into my diets, I can determine exactly which are the biggest culprits or triggers based on the level of comfort or discomfort I feel. Perhaps the biggest adjustment is eating only one solid meal a day—at lunchtime. For breakfast and dinner, this approach calls for a smoothie, soup, or juice.

Junger recommends that the initial three weeks of the *Clean* detox program encompass a quiet time with reflection, emotional detoxing, and moderate movement that all benefit the process. Limiting strenuous exercise is key because energy levels, calorie intake, and bodily priorities need to stay focused on the detoxification process. As the body readjusts to its natural, healthy body mass, an unexpected bonus is losing weight.

MY PERSONAL STARTING POINT

Despite talking the talk about my newfound interest in health and longevity, changing my lifestyle proved challenging. I was still overeating and overdrinking. I'd managed to keep active and swim, walk, or practice yoga regularly—activities partially to compensate for my persistent overindulgence and keep from becoming overweight.

Yet committing to a detox program was such a massive departure—too "over the top," too unconventional—that I resisted. Maintaining my regular family, social, and work life didn't allow for that. At the same time, I felt drawn to take a big leap. Then a serendipitous window opened. My daughters and wife went to Africa to visit her mother for a few weeks, and I had to stay behind to start a new business in London. With time on my own and nothing to do but work, I gave the *Clean* program a try.

First Step: The Elimination Diet

The program recommended starting a few days earlier than the actual protocol on tackling the elimination diet—that is, avoiding all foods that might cause the body any possible immune system activation. This allows the immune system to focus on beginning to deep clean the body and not fighting any incoming threats. The list of foods to avoid is long, and the author of *Clean* reviews the reasons to temporarily eliminate each one. For these three weeks, sticking to the general protocol is recommended. Any occasional lapse should be countered by resuming the program—and not feeling guilty.

My first step was to remove all restricted foods from my cupboards and refrigerator to stop me from impulsively opening them to see what's there. I've never been partial to processed and prepared foods, so taking those away wasn't a problem. The same went for pasta, sugar, and most sweets. Then I emptied or put away my liquor bottles, gave a few bottles of wine to friends, and locked the wine cellar.

The First Few Days

The novelty of the first few days—and feeling my different reactions—made this cleanse an adventure. The smoothies, soups, and liquid meals for breakfast and dinner challenged me because I wanted that feeling of being full at dinner. Dr. Junger warned about this—that the body and psyche will put up all sorts of resistance to bail out. Yet this is something I've found happens with every positive step I've taken in pursuing a healthier life. (More on the persistence of resistance to come.)

Also, my energy levels were all over the place. Headaches were common during these days as well, which is acknowledged to be a quickly passing phase. I decided to buy the ingredients for my one fresh meal daily to make it an adventure. I looked forward to that meal every day, partially out of hunger, but mostly due to the pleasure of finding and preparing what was truly good for me.

I knew alcohol would be a problem, given that a few big drinks or glasses of wine had become a nightly ritual in my adult years. I was eager to take a break from that, but I knew it would be hard.

Sticking with It All

My first and probably most important lesson was to commit to something and come out the other end—the only way to see if a practice works for me. Giving up at the first sign of resistance or discomfort, or not starting at all, was the easy, comfortable way of not learning and changing. It would also keep me from getting any benefit out of something potentially good for me. Without the warnings and stories from previous followers in the *Clean* book, as well as hearing about the benefits they enjoyed afterward, I might have talked myself into stopping for a host of reasons.

Also, I found that saying things like, "So you would rather die a few years earlier than stick this out for three weeks and see if it works?" That helped! Luckily for me, the first few days, as difficult as they were, weren't tough enough to pull me off the program. Any resistance faded quickly as I began to feel the benefits.

WHY A DETOX WORKS: HUNGER AND TIME

For the detox process to work, it's essential to give our bodies long periods of noneating. There's no getting around it. Part of why a detox works is by being hungry, which requires getting used to. Fasts are a time-honored cultural practice to improve not only our health but our spirit life. When the body isn't doing something it prioritizes above cleaning and detox—such as sex, digestion, fear of danger, even exercise, work, or just business—it goes back to housekeeping. When we're engaged in other priorities, the "background" immunity housekeeping goes into low gear. It operates at its highest levels during sleep, followed by low-level movement that's enjoyable and nonstressful.

In modern life, we're used to thinking hunger is bad and needs to be addressed immediately. However, for millions of years, humans lived with hunger as a regular sensation daily. Even when food was abundant, our ancestors didn't overeat, something we know from modern hunter-gatherer studies. Modern schedules simply do not afford enough time for detoxification to kick in since it takes six to eight hours to fully digest a meal. During that time, the body's main priority is not housekeeping but digestion.

For this reason, Junger, in *Clean*, recommends at least a twelve-hour break from eating daily, even after finishing the detox program. This means a small early dinner and *no* evening snacking. Smoothies and soups reduce the usual time your body takes to digest a meal from six to eight hours down to two to four hours. These forms allow your body to get back to detoxing and healing sooner.

When I don't put anything in my body that takes extra work to eliminate or detoxify (such as alcohol, sugar, caffeine, and prepared foods), I ensure my immune system gets more time and energy to work. When I eat toxic foods, my immune system tends to surround and neutralize toxins with mucous and white blood cells to eliminate immediate danger, and then to "park" those cells for removal later. Many times, it never comes back to those parked cells, and their presence can cause disease. An intense detox program allows for a *deep* clean, like cleaning out neglected closets and drawers.

Toxins in the affected cells can turn deadly. Using blood tests on many subjects, Dr. Junger calculates a three-week timetable as the amount of time to get to a detoxification level that's closer to the way our bodies are meant to be. The bottom line: *Everything works better without accumulated sludge in our bodies.*

THE JOY OF EMPTINESS

My body welcomed the feeling of not being full. Instead, I experienced a new lightness while feeling adequately fueled and energetic. I realized overeating is a major cause of lethargy and low energy. The hungry sensation I felt became a pleasant sensation instead of a reason to run to the refrigerator. Yes, I had been eating out of boredom as much as need.

In fact, with less food, my energy levels increased dramatically. I felt buzzed and vibrant, as if the emptiness was attracting new ideas and insights. And I was ready for them! This lightness was the opposite of light-headedness or weakness. I felt as if a new internal spaciousness had been opened within me, both physically and emotionally. I discovered resources that had been previously hidden from my sight.

THE ROLE OF REAL HUNGER

In evolving from ape to man, the human body's primary energy revolution was being able to go hungry for long periods. Our ancestors thrived by being able to hunt and forage for food, probably eating little bits along the way. And besides, becoming full and gluttonously lethargic would have meant one thing: an increased likelihood of injury or death by predators or enemies. Low alertness and energy levels were ingredients for danger. More important to survival than relishing a big meal was staying active, alert, and wary. They had to have their wits about them and be ready to spring into action. At that time, the human body was probably more sensitive to being "full" than it is now. Cavemen didn't have the enormous bellies and other fat stores common in people today.

"Hungry" means slightly depleted but not starving, and it's historically more natural to us than its opposite. Our bodies learn to like that sensation once we wean ourselves off ritual eating. These days, we pay dearly for slumping on the sofa in front of the TV in a state of utter fullness.

During my detox, I started being "comfortably empty" yet nutritionally satiated. What a revelation! Less food but of better quality gave me more energy than before, along with a steadier mood and outlook. I also realized that eating three big meals a day, while probably necessary for children, has become more of a social and workplace accommodation than a necessity for adults.

MOVEMENT DURING DETOX

As far as exercise went, I made sure to walk or bike more than usual every day, plus do gentle yoga. Yet I didn't push or exhaust myself. Mostly, I didn't allow myself to get distracted from my body's priority: detoxing as it related to my central mission of health and longevity.

I remained conscious of the detox process throughout the three weeks. Becoming more appreciative of my body, cleaning things out, and liking my lighter self topped a long list of revelations. An attuned awareness of my body became a critically important characteristic that has stuck with me over the years and become amplified as I continue to learn.

TIME OF REFLECTION

I spent a lot of time reflecting about my prospects for a future healthy life in old age. Those positive mental and emotional aspects—what Dr. Junger calls Quantum Detox—are a big part of why detoxes have become popular. Healthy diet goes hand in hand with having a healthy mind and spirit. We can clean out subterranean emotional baggage as well as physical toxins during a cleanse. Cleaning up my soul and messy inner life is where I eventually headed. Yet my expanded awareness of the link between my physical and emotional life began during this time of reflection.

Here are eight observations I made during detox:

1. **No more blocked nose and sinuses.** These had chronically been blocked and stuffy, especially at night, but they completely cleared with detoxifying. Experimenting after the detox program, I slowly went back to regular eating, one food group at a time, to see which foods had different effects. I discovered that my blocked nose condition related to eating wheat and flour as well as sugar and alcohol. By adjusting my diet to avoid these foods, I've been able to stay mainly congestion free.
2. **Reduced joint stiffness.** I'd had stiffness historically in my hands as well as in my lower back and hips. The detox significantly reduced this stiffness. I attribute this to the absence of sugar and alcohol as well as the general level of cleaning my body was going through.
3. **Improved digestion.** Feelings of bloating and fullness went away. I learned later that these first three symptoms are linked with inflammation, a major factor in disease and aging discussed in the introduction to Part II. My detox protocol dramatically reduced the low-level chronic inflammation in my body.
4. **Decreased appetite.** Not only did my appetite *not* increase, it decreased or went away most of the time to the point of not wanting to have my evening soup or smoothie. The author of *Clean* warns readers not to skip these meals, though. If one's nutrition levels are too low, the liver won't be able to filter the harmful toxins the body has started to release into the bloodstream.
5. **Rapid weight loss.** During the three weeks of detox, I lost about fifteen pounds. At six feet tall and 175 pounds, I wasn't

exactly heavy, but by the end of three weeks, I weighed 160 pounds, felt lighter, and had more energy. I also lost most of my stomach belly. When my daughters returned from their trip, they seem amazed and happy about this. (I stabilized at around 165 pounds and have stayed that way.)
6. **Discovery of probiotics.** "Probiotic" refers to the bacteria that inhabit our colon and enable us to process food. I started to take a probiotic supplement during the detox.
7. **Calorie restriction (CR) and intermittent fasting (IF)**. These are strategies to combat aging. The author of *Clean* helped me see how these digestive helpers make my body more efficient, resilient, and able to renew itself.
8. **Reset my baseline of optimum health**. I treasure the vitality I experience in having vast and beneficial health effects happen inside me. I knew this approach could only enhance my plan to live longer and stay healthy.

SELECTIVE GATEKEEPER

One of the wonderful things to know is that every one of the one hundred trillion cells in my body knows whether a cell is ONE OF US or NOT US. The creation of life came with this crucial distinction—from the first cell or bacteria defined as "alive" to our ultracomplex selves. This quality of separateness is also the essence of how the immune system works. It's a highly selective gatekeeper, allowing entry only to helpful friends (ONE OF US) and keeping out or neutralizing dangerous, potential enemies (NOT US). What a revelation—to realize this whole immune system was ceaselessly protecting me.

"Given that, how can I enhance my immune system to be a big part of my evolving health program?" I asked myself.

Feeling energetic on less food opened my eyes about how my

body responded when diverted from my regular eating and drinking habits. As the effects of lifestyle on health and longevity became obvious, I questioned whether the "good life" of eating and drinking, especially for celebrations, was the *actual* reason behind the lethargy and many chronic conditions seen today.

More questions surfaced. How would I be able to manage all of this, to square that circle? Would I have to live this way all the time? How far was I willing to commit to my health and longevity project? Just how serious was I about maintaining my health and keeping the promise I had made to myself and my daughters? Did it mean changing my lifestyle in a major way, particularly around social drinking and eating?

I'm not alone with my doubts. The resistance most people display when I suggest doing a detox is staggering. They say, "I couldn't do that. Three weeks is too long. I would miss my evening meal too much. I enjoy what I like to eat, and that's that."

I see how we can get fixated in our eating routines and tastes by deep bonds that largely stay unexamined. It's as if our taste buds have minds of their own separate from what we *know* is good for us.

WHAT I LEARNED FROM DETOXIFYING

Here's what I learned from my detox experience: *What I ate, when I ate, and when I didn't eat had a dramatic effect on the way I felt and what I thought.* My old way of eating was inhibiting my body's natural ability to heal itself. After the detox, I could only project that my body was healthier because I felt more energetic and carried less weight. I felt more optimistic as well, particularly about accomplishing what I had set out to do. That encouraged me to look forward to other aspects of pursuing my health goals.

The word "health" stems from the old English or Germanic word for "whole," meaning "sound" and "complete." The word "heal" means "to recover or to restore to health, to become whole again." It's the active, dynamic process our bodies are born with, a priceless gift from the universe. Our bodies *want* to heal; they're programmed to stay whole and healthy, to continue to thrive.

I realized the answers to this riddle lay within me, as much in my psyche as in my physical body. My unhealthy habits had their source in my mind and my beliefs. I realized there's no shortcut to uncovering the truth by reading about others' experiences, nor will trusting what they say fill the bill. *The only truth is what resonates inside from actual practice.*

However, my detox experience raised a giant question. If my appetite couldn't be trusted to guide me with eating and diet, then the same principle had to apply to exercise, lifestyle, and all the health practices I had been investigating. A budding sense of what constitutes *truth* about health and what *doesn't* began at this time. Again, the only way to answer my questions came from adopting new practices and seeing what would happen. Finding ways to measure and judge the effectiveness of my actions beyond how they made me feel, though, would prove challenging.

I ended my detoxification program feeling remarkably healthy, energized, empowered, and challenged to do even more. I had begun to see what my eventual food plan would consist of for a healthy and long life (outlined in Part II). Although I recognized I had much to learn, I'd still taken that first step, engaged in the effort, and finished with a highly positive outcome. The stakes were too high *not* to continue. After all, I was getting healthy both for my life and for the lives of my children. *Nothing* could be more important.

3

Four Doctors

"Physician, heal thyself: then wilt thou also heal thy patient. Let it be his best cure to see with his eyes him who maketh himself whole."
—JESUS OF NAZARETH

*"I will prevent disease whenever I can,
for prevention is preferable to cure."*
—EXCERPT FROM HIPPOCRATIC OATH, MODERN VERSION

My detox experience gave me a level of health I wanted to sustain and expand, so I scheduled visits with a few doctors to see what their advice held for me. I planned to ask each of them one simple question: "What can I do to increase my health and longevity?"

I also wanted a medical checkup and tests to see what the professionals look for in someone my age. I was more interested in proactive advice—what could be done to *prevent* disease as opposed to someday reacting to an already present one. What would they recommend for lifestyle, diet, and exercise to improve my energy, health, and longevity? What personalized advice could I get that targeted concerns to watch out for? My findings proved to be revelatory and unexpected.

I selected four doctors from the four corners of my life. I lived in London at that time but had spent most of my life in New York where my traditional go-to doctor lived. I found a traditional MD in London whom I liked. Sensing that some answers might lie in less traditional directions, I also chose two alternative doctors, MDs as well, one in New York and one in London.

DEFINING MY GOALS

My goal was to avoid any kind of chronic medical condition or use of pharmaceuticals commonly used by older people. When people start that kind of care, whether it be prescriptions, surgery, or other treatments, I observed their quality of life decline, sometimes precipitously. The same was true due to falls and accidents as well as traumatic events such as the loss of a spouse. I believe exceptions occur when people use their conditions as a wake-up call and do more prevention practices.

Maybe a decline was brought on by thinking that, when something was wrong, they were being treated and therefore felt they *must* be sick. Or perhaps the side effects of their drugs was a factor. To me, the big slippery slope was one I'd do my best to avoid for as long as possible. My ultimate goal? Maintaining or increasing my full complement of physical and mental faculties.

Imprinted in me was having seen both my parents and grandparents get cancer and start treatment. (Luckily, my adoption at birth distanced me from *that* gene pool. More on this in chapter 20, Genes.) In each case, I saw each of these relatives begin a slide that didn't last long. After a slight temporary reprieve, none of them ever got well enough to fully live again. I wanted to avoid getting sick in the first place.

What follows is a summary of what my research revealed. I have changed some of the descriptions of the doctors to protect their identities. Yet, in sharing these stories, I'm emphasizing how important developing my individual health plan—including listening to my "inner doctor"—became.

DOCTOR ONE

The first doctor I saw was a functional medicine doctor and detox specialist. I reported the details of my *Clean* detox to her and what had happened. She was pleased to hear it had worked so well. She took time to explain her own journey through conventional medicine and how she had become frustrated with only *treating* and not *preventing* disease.

I instinctively liked and trusted this doctor. She was passionate in her advice about dietary health, the benefits of limiting intake of food, and avoiding processed foods. She looked and acted like she followed the advice herself. I filled her in on my health mission and asked, "What advice can you give me to help me do that?"

I had told her I was adopted at birth and both my birth parents had died young from cancer, so my genetic history remained a mystery. She said that whatever genes I possessed, I was lucky not to have those of my birth parents. She recommended a slightly different program of detoxing and suggested I read books such as *Blue Zones* and *Healthy at 100*, describing societies reputed for their people's longevity.

My Health and Drinking

We covered details about my heart and my drinking. I told her I'd been diagnosed with a heart murmur early in life, but it had never stopped me from doing anything. Today, it was almost unnoticeable. From my blood test results, she saw my heart panels were favorable:

low overall cholesterol, high HDL, and low inflammation. She listened to my heart and said the murmur was slight but would recommend a stress echocardiogram or scan for more information.

She also asked what I instinctively felt represented the biggest threat to my health. My drinking, I responded, which I told her was out of control. Based on my reading, over time alcohol would represent the biggest threat to my health. I had felt great on the *Clean* program without the alcohol, but I had gone back to drinking shortly after, as though I'd never detoxed. When she asked why I drank so much, I said, "Mainly out of shyness and feeling awkward in social situations." Alcohol gave me confidence and relaxed me.

Then she asked this pointed question: "I thought you said you would do anything for your daughters. ANYTHING. This is something you need to do—for them as much as yourself. Because you are right. Alcohol *will* affect your health at some point. We can't predict how or when, but chances are it could severely damage both the length and quality of your life." Her remarks made a deep impression on me. They started a process that dragged on inside me before being resolved.

Needed Blood Tests

When I asked what she'd look for in my profile, she gave me an extensive list of different blood tests I should have regularly—more extensive than I'd thought—that included minerals, vitamins, and inflammation tests. These markers could show if something was out of sync and indicate future problems. I got these tests about six months later, and she reviewed them for me, then gave me a clean bill of health with no warnings or specific areas of concern.

Because my detox results were so profound, I instinctively agreed to the health approach she suggested. She combined traditional Western medicine with its laser-like ability to intervene and diagnose with older but equally wise methods of prevention like fasting and eating only natural foods. I did feel uncomfortable that her advice only related to food. It didn't cover other areas such as exercise and emotional factors. I instinctively knew staying healthy in my later years had to involve more than nutrition.

Blind Trust in Doctors

Shortly after meeting her, I realized I'd developed an almost blind trust in doctors since childhood. I'd never seen them as people with their own subjective opinions and personalities. As a child, I regarded a doctor as possessing the power to dispense healing, making him or her the closest thing to God. I believed that, because certain people were doctors, they could and should be listened to. People in my family also believed we should never ignore doctors' instructions or disagree with them.

These beliefs make sad statements about our lack of medical knowledge as well as our lack of responsibility for taking care of our own health. This visit in my early sixties was the beginning of taking health into my own hands and diverging from my traditional doctor-centered definition of health. Relying on my own feelings and knowledge to guide my health—rather than "trusting the doctor"—became a big part of my journey.

DOCTOR TWO

The second doctor had been my personal physician for more than ten years in Lower Manhattan. His office was in the lower floor of a

Greenwich Village brownstone near where I used to live. He and his family lived upstairs in the rest of the building.

An avid believer in interventionist medicine (what Western medicine is best at) and a phenomenal diagnostician when something is wrong, he had never given me advice about prevention. That being said, he was someone who had never rushed any check-up or consultation.

I asked him what I could do to foster an active, healthy life in my later years. My regular check-up with him came around my sixtieth birthday, so he had my charts, history, and blood test results in front of him. His first reaction? As he looked at the charts, he said, "Let me see what we think is going to get you." Then he said, "Heart is good, no signs of any cancers. Anyway, you don't know your genes because of the adoption, so we can't predict any likelihood. I'd say you are healthy, fit, and active. Although it's fine now, maybe your prostate, so make sure you get your PSA tested regularly. Maybe colon cancer because you had a benign polyp removed on your last colonoscopy, so do that regularly or even increase the frequency. Other than that, stay tuned and come in if anything is bothering you."

Quality-of-Life Issues

Then I asked him about my drinking. He turned it back on me, inquiring how much I drank. At least a half bottle of wine every night and usually either more wine or wine *and* a predinner hard drink or two, I answered. He said I should cut down. Or if I couldn't do that, then I should quit. He also recommended Alcoholics Anonymous if I found quitting hard to do, confirming my drinking came with a genuine risk of complications or disease in the future. He also pointed out quality-of-life issues that accompany drinking too much, adding, "The lowest-risk path would be to stop."

I asked if exercise and diet mattered. He replied by saying whatever I liked eating was fine. I should exercise if I felt like it, but in the long run, he didn't think those things made much difference to one's longevity. "If we knew more about your genes, it would give us a better picture of what to watch out for," he replied. This doctor seemed resigned to my having a disease coming out of nowhere and "getting me" with little cause or effect from lifestyle. According to him, what mattered most was having a good doctor to treat me when something happened.

At this point, let me say the doctor, in his fifties, had gotten a bit overweight himself. I've always believed doctors should be examples of health to their patients through their own lifestyles. This view may be a stretch, I know, but it was how I felt. On the flip side, lots of health peddlers look and act great just to sell you something.

I knew Doctor Two played golf on weekends, but otherwise he was fairly sedentary. And I knew a number of his patients who were also overweight. He lived among, and catered to, an affluent crowd who all lived the same sort of lifestyle. A house in the Hamptons, eating out at top restaurants, and entertaining all the time (like I used to do) were the norm in this set. Although I had once been part of that world, it now seemed conventional and uninformed. My independence from fitting into that world was also a budding part of the journey I was on.

The Detox Question

When I mentioned my detox and other health aspects I was working on to improve and extend my life, Doctor Two became paternal and somewhat dismissive. He said that if they made me feel better, I should do them but cautioned me not to go overboard. "These things are fads and could be dangerous," he said quietly, going strictly by Western medicine's model for a modern lifestyle.

However, a part of him "got" where I was headed about detoxing. I told him my lower back and hips had been bothering me (as they had on and off for most of my life). The former stiffness had thankfully gone away when I did the detox. "Really?" he said, without giving much credit to the subsequent change. "Here's something else that might help." He then gave me the name and number of someone who he himself used for his own bad back—a personal trainer and physical therapist.

I did see the person he recommended several times. As it turned out, he was steeped in traditional yoga practice and adapted positions into studio-based movement and Pilates routines. I still incorporate what I learned into my daily fifteen- to thirty-minute morning stretching, strength, and gratitude routine in addition to my regular workout. Of all the medical advice I've received from this doctor, this last proactive piece affected me most deeply in a long-lasting way—something he had offered off the cuff.

When I told Doctor Two about my back problem, I half expected to be given a prescription for a muscle relaxer or anti-inflammatory. Instead, he gave me this referral, knowing I was likely to embrace it over medicine. And I think, in his heart of hearts, he knew his advice was not only better for me personally, but I'd be more amenable to *accepting* it, given who I was. That's the sign of understanding that the kind of treatment patients will follow depends on their individuality. Unless something is life-threatening and needs forceful intervention, most people simply do what they feel comfortable with rather than willingly change major habits or beliefs to find a healthier path. He realized I'd be most open to an active, physical approach for my back problems, and he was spot-on in doing so.

High Marks, but . . .

If I'm ever sick with a disease requiring interventionist Western medical care, I would like a doctor like this to treat me. He's an excellent diagnostician with up-to-date research and an array of treatments available. He's connected to the best hospitals. Also, he's someone I can talk to, work with, and respect. I know he would listen if I objected to something he proposed. Yet I walked out of his office with the distinct impression that, as far as preventive health was concerned, he wouldn't be nearly as useful.

My conclusion after these two doctor visits: *Prevention isn't on the radar for most traditional doctors.*

DOCTOR THREE

I'd seen a highly recommended private doctor while spending time in London. His service was in addition to the National Health Service, a universal British medical resource. Doctor Three was a bit of a gadfly who embodied the essence of British quirkiness. That trait can be as entertaining as it is frustrating, especially if one's goal is to get something done efficiently and thoroughly.

I've found that most professional advice in England, whether in medicine, law, or accounting, is so convoluted and wrapped up in manners, tradition, and image that the core gets hidden in the process. I miss the "cut to the chase" attitude I'm used to from New Yorkers. By comparison, the British don't want to stick their necks out to be direct, so advice gets paved over with verbiage like "it could be this, but it also could be that." Some of it is surely to cover their asses and appear to be right no matter what.

Armed with my ever-increasing knowledge, I went to Doctor Three for an enhanced panel of blood tests. These had been recommended by Doctor One, the detox doctor, as supplements to my regular blood panels. This doctor immediately looked askance at the additional tests, saying they weren't necessary and were a waste of money. However, he would do them if I *really* wanted them. I said I did want them, and I explained my whole program.

Point blank I asked what he would recommend overall for a longer, healthier life. His response was succinct: "Eat, drink, and be merry." In short, Doctor Three told me nothing could be done. I heard every cliché about older age on earth from him. "It's all in your genes." "You could be hit by a bus tomorrow." "Enjoy what time you have left."

There's an element of wisdom in these hackneyed sayings, but not in this context. For example, when I asked about the wisdom of exercise, he claimed nothing has been proven. He did acknowledge that movement was important, adding that, for him, movement meant gardening, but only on weekends. The same applied to diet. "Eat what you enjoy. No restrictions." When I asked him about alcohol and my level of drinking, he told me to spend as much as I was currently spending on alcohol but buy the best quality wines so I would drink less that way.

I wasn't surprised to discover Doctor Three spent his vacation time in France and Europe eating gourmet food and drinking fine wines. The advice he gave me was the advice he was living himself. The self-justification seemed obvious; I've seen too many other people use this type of rationale.

Don't get me wrong. I have no qualms with Doctor Three as a physician for regular medical conditions. When it comes to interventionist medicine, he has enormous knowledge of disease and medicine. But once again, in terms of prevention, little substantial advice was coming from the traditional medical community.

PREVENTION AT A LOW PREMIUM

Traditional doctors show resistance to practices like detoxing, healthy diets, and plentiful exercise. The conventional way was based on how they were trained and how they've lived. Yet it was so contrary to what my own sensations and my gut were telling me—both of which I was trusting more and more.

Here's one final word on Doctor Three or, rather, the view of life in England as compared with the USA: While not a monopoly, a belief in traditional, old-fashioned remedies and wives' tales is still widespread in England. I've found the culture to be distrustful of most new ideas, especially anything that would cause someone to change. While maintaining a certain amount of cynicism toward every new theory of health and medicine that comes along may be wise, British doctors' wholesale dismissal of newness and the reversion to "doctor knows best" dominate.

What did my exercise with these doctors show me? That they are real people who simply hold different views. I could take their advice—or not. Any curiosity people have about their health (and certainly the irrepressible curiosity I had about mine) deserves to have maximum light shone on it and followed.

REVOLUTIONARY CHANGES

We're living in an age of revolutionary changes in health. These include not only *how* it's provided, but *what* information and resources are available. In reality, one's health is based not only on preventive practices like those I was pursuing but on full-scale democratization.

People *do* want to take greater control of their own health decisions. I know the arena of self-care can be tricky in the age of Dr. Google. But by telling my story, I want to impress upon people how they can grapple with self-health as I have.

I've learned that real knowledge could be attained only through traveling a path of action. The most potent knowledge is based on experience and emotion, not thought. And a desire for deeper knowledge of health has beckoned me to take action.

DOCTOR FOUR

The fourth doctor I saw was an acupuncturist in London and a practicing Buddhist. A certified medical doctor, he was trained in both Eastern and Western medicine but hadn't practiced Western medicine in years. He turned to acupuncture because he felt he could do more to influence his patients' health that way than through conventional practices. Much like Doctor One, he was fed up with simply treating disease and its symptoms while feeling helpless about preventing it in the first place.

A Different Approach

Right off the bat, Doctor Four and I talked before doing any treatment or diagnosis. How refreshing! I told him what I was doing and shared my medical history. He wrote it all down and then simply asked, "How do you feel?"

"Right now?"

"Yes," he said. "Right now, how do you feel?"

"Fine," I replied. "No obvious problems. But aren't you supposed to check me over and tell me if I'm okay or not?"

"That's not how it works in my kind of medicine. People can't lie when they try to answer that simple question. It's too obvious an answer. And if they lie outwardly, they know inside they're doing it. The truth will make itself known to them somehow. It's in answering this question that people determine what they need me for. I can confirm or deny what they're feeling, but it all starts with them knowing how they feel. For instance, you said, 'No obvious problems.' Are there any *unobvious* problems?" he asked.

"I think I'm drinking too much alcohol, and it will eventually affect my health," I said in response.

"Okay, that's better. Now let me check you over."

Acupuncture Treatment

Acupuncture is based on three pulse levels that a skilled practitioner can feel at once. How weak or strong each pulse is and how balanced they are with each other make up the essence of a practitioner's diagnosis. Each pulse represents a different system in the body—the liver, heart, and kidney pulses. In Chinese medicine, they consist of systems that cover the whole body and are roughly the equivalent of the neurological, endocrine, and immune systems. They need to be in balance with each other and have enough power to all work harmoniously. If the systems are out of balance, energy flows start causing unhealthy responses in the body.

Also, acupuncture does not distinguish between physical and emotional aspects of health. Doctor Four told me that links between these two aspects of health are encouraged, as they have power over each other. Again, balance is important. By stimulating meridians and points in the body with shallow needles, acupuncture aims to restore this balance when they get out of kilter.

The meridians and points are not actual physical structures that can be seen by X-ray, scan, or surgery. However, new CT scans claim it can "see" them via increased oxygen levels while ultrasensitive electrical measurements claim increased microvoltages. Some are the same system of sensitive pressure points that provide relief when stimulated and are used in all kinds of massage—from Swedish to Shiatsu. They are also the same channels of energy that yoga and myofascial muscle work are based on. These practices are part of an Eastern healing spectrum in which massive health wisdom lies.

I lay down on the treatment table in Doctor Four's office after removing my shirt, shoes, and socks. He took my pulse with three fingers. I felt like he was playing a tune on a trumpet, pressing down on each point in slightly different combinations. He said my liver pulse was indeed weak but that my other systems appeared normal.

He proceeded to rebalance my whole body but warned me that something had caused it to get out of balance in the first place. He inserted ten or fifteen or so different microthin needles up to two centimeters deep at points on my feet, leg, stomach, ear, head, and shoulders. He put them in quickly and painlessly with a twirling motion. He then took my pulse again and said, "Good. All in balance now. I'm going to leave you like this for a little while."

After he left the semidarkened room, I lay quietly for thirty minutes or so. When he returned, he took my pulse again and removed the needles. He asked me to return in two weeks to see how long the treatment had lasted and how I was feeling. From there, we could make a plan.

I must admit, a certain amount of "unscientific" and nonprovable theory was involved in this treatment, though some of it made a lot of sense. I was particularly taken by his asking how I felt and saying I couldn't fool myself on this question. I've heard that, in the Far East, doctors are paid for keeping their patients well and giving advice about how to *not* get sick—both physically and emotionally. If patients do get sick, they stop paying the doctor until they are better. Is this actually happening? I don't know, but the whole notion of prevention strikes me as a big wake-up call for Western medicine to take notice.

I asked Doctor Four my stock question: "What can I do to stay healthy and live as long as possible?" His reply was to practice what seemed "sensible" to me. He said that how I feel about whatever I practice is as important as the practice itself, and to use my internal guidance system to judge what was good for me, not to simply follow advice. He said I would uncover many practices in my research, but the ones that made sense to me—that I embraced and felt connected to—were the ones that would provide the best foundation.

My biggest takeaway between Western and Eastern medicine was the profound difference between them. The Eastern view centers on interconnectedness, patience, and attention as its foundation. The entire body and mind, as well as what we think and feel about them, are a complete system, with no aspect functioning independently as in Western medicine. Nothing could be treated without addressing the balance and harmony of the whole organism. Western medicine tends to treat the body as being made up of separate parts. Any dysfunction in those parts is targeted and treated as it arises.

The organic systems that make up our bodies constantly interact with the world around them, with a flow of energy, nutrients, toxins, air, emotions, and other elements being exchanged, shared, or repulsed constantly. Acupuncture acknowledges that it takes time to heal and rebalance. While Western treatments might quiet the symptoms, people can't get completely healthy with quick results from a pill or injection.

I continued treatment with Doctor Four for a few more sessions, then went back to see him many years later and still do on occasion. I'm practicing such a robust health plan that he tells me, "Whatever you're doing, keep it up."

TAKEAWAYS ABOUT THE FOUR DOCTORS

In terms of specific answers or advice I sought in these doctor visits, I learned less than I had anticipated. The absence of prevention advice marked my biggest takeaway. Maybe the norm of aging is so prevalent, no widespread results are available for what I was searching for. Asking for extended years of high-quality life in later years seemed elusive in the traditional medical community. I felt disappointed, yet was spurred to keep searching for answers. Increasingly, I sensed these answers resided as much *inside* me as on the outside.

In visiting the four doctors, I sought advice about keeping me from *getting* sick and helping me *stay* energetic and healthy. Doctor One came closest to addressing my request, and Doctor Four showed me aspects of health that were new to me. The two traditional doctors provided almost no help in this regard.

However, I know this way of practicing medicine separately is shifting as functional and integrative medicine gains ground. Traditional doctors are acknowledging the benefits of exercise and diet more, with studies backing up these views. (See Bibliography.)

These visits marked the beginning of my own self-health management, a way of life that turns to doctors as resources but not supreme authorities. Ultimately, I had to put responsibility for my health squarely on myself by following my inspiration and gut feelings—just as I had experienced on that New Jersey train. I realized this journey might be lonelier than I thought.

4

Born to Move

"Exercise six days a week for the rest of your life."
—HARRY'S FIRST RULE, *Younger Next Year*

*"A body in motion tends to stay in motion.
A body at rest tends to stay at rest."*
—ISAAC NEWTON

From everything I read, movement needed to play a central role in my emerging longevity plan. The doctors I had visited didn't mention it, even though the health benefits of different sorts of movement and exercise were obvious and seemed instinctually "right." In addition to physical benefits, moving has also made me feel better. My visceral reconnection to it, fueled by endorphins and self-satisfaction, has always positively affected my mood.

I was no stranger to gyms, pools, or yoga mats. I'd been doing one exercise or another for over twenty years. Since my midthirties, movement had been a way of dealing with stress, overeating, and overdrinking. Plus, it helped me look fit and attractive. These benefits were palpable and somewhat addictive. As part of the package that defined "who I was," movement also fed the image of "how I'm seen." I liked how it *felt* to be fit, strong, and energetic. My top four exercise choices? Swimming, yoga, walking, and biking.

TRANSFORMED MY APPROACH

However, my awakening on the train ride to New Jersey that I discussed in chapter 1 transformed how I approached movement. I had never before cared about the tangible health benefits of exercise. Like many who work out regularly, getting fit and looking good in the mirror prevailed over health aims. Appearance and attractiveness—external, not internal—had been my primary goals.

This was also true with eating and drinking; I'd binge after a workout, believing I could indulge in both without feeling the consequences. But since my detox, I learned that weight loss comes from factors other than exercise. What passes for "working out" in modern life is not the same as maintaining my health and mobility as I got older.

The book *Younger Next Year* by Chris Crowley and Dr. Harry Lodge became my initial exercise bible. Mainly, it advocated the benefits of regular aerobics and movement in later life, and it featured both medical and evolutionary backup for its findings. The text provided strength and lifestyle advice as well.

With this book's outline as my guide, I began going to the gym. Crowley and Lodge's first piece of advice was to use a heart monitor to gauge my level of aerobic activity, something I'd never done. But that introduced me to target exertion zones, which has shaped how I've approached movement and exercise ever since.

WHAT OUR BODIES WERE MADE FOR

For most people, daily movement is taken for granted. Nature has been working on how humans move for billions of years and especially on their exquisitely intricate ability to move on two legs.

Going back to the first single-celled organisms of our evolutionary ancestors, movement evolved from our need to find food and avoid danger. It has since developed into the complex and varied forms seen in nature today—from crawling to walking to swimming to flying.

During the millions of years it took to evolve into a walking upright posture and using our arms and hands, foraging and hunting took up most of our waking time. The goals advocated in *Younger Next Year* have simply mimicked the same activities our evolutionary ancestors did. The countless types and intensities of movements involved in walking, running, hunting, throwing, fighting, digging, pulling, and climbing led to our bodies possessing the myriad range and forces of motion they have now. *We were made this way.* Today, our bodies still crave this kind of activity, which requires us to be healthy and well balanced. What better guide to maintaining our bodies well into later life than using nature's own formula?

In contrast, humans have aspired to seek comfort and ease only in recent history. These modern trends are driven by social values and are primarily related to status and image. But these changes come at a great price to our continued ability to move. I shudder to think what our bodies are becoming because of our sedentary lives, a process that anthropologist Daniel Lieberman, in his book *The Story of the Human Body*, called *dis-evolution*.

As I was to learn, this trend doesn't apply to movement alone but to many aspects of modern life. Our ancestors had to constantly move, struggle, work, and fight throughout their days. They were in continual, direct contact with the power and wonder of nature with few "taking it easy" breaks. After all, the slowest runner gets caught by the lion.

OUR BODIES LONG FOR MOVEMENT

Our bodies respond to a longing for movement by getting more agile and gaining strength. They're built for the grueling challenges humans faced on the African plain. Under the harshest conditions, we became strong, tough, and smart enough to survive. This is the true miracle of our current existence, one that we're ready to discard on the altar of "taking it easy." God forbid, we have to walk a few blocks or carry something heavy. "What a pain!" we protest.

A need for high energy and strenuous movement allowed our bodies to evolve—and we still have that evolutionary memory in our bones. We developed strength and endurance by overcoming the harsh challenges of prehistoric times. The exercise the authors advocate in *Younger Next Year* aims to recapture this inner power, with "modern exercise" copying this process. That means when we get tired and expend effort, we break down muscle and circulate blood. This sets off a chain of biochemical reactions to rebuild and heal, allowing us to be stronger than before.

That process begins with fatigue. We tire ourselves out when we push ourselves, which then makes us feel relaxed. Nature provides that perk to us as a gift. How cool is that? While that capacity lessens as we get older, still, we have more of it inside than we're led to believe. Plenty of tales have been told of those who found the energy to stay athletically active into their eighties, nineties, and even longer. I committed to be one of them.

TWO BASIC SPEEDS

Using a heart monitor as my guide, I began to exercise at two basic speeds—"long and even" and "short and fast," with long and even taking up most of my time. Even does not mean slow. It means active and elevated but comfortable, able to carry on a conversation or not feel exertion while moving. My heart rate measures in the range of 50 to 65 percent of my maximum target heart rate (usually measured as 220 minus one's age, with 180 minus your age as another metric for calculating aerobic zone heart rate). This range is referred to as "aerobic," which signifies oxygen is being used.

Short and fast means just what it says: exertion happens in short bursts above 75 percent of the maximum target heart rate. This is referred to as the anaerobic range when the body's exertion exceeds the rate at which oxygen can be supplied to the muscles. The anaerobic system kicks in, used in short bursts for situations of danger or need, like hunting and fighting. In prehistoric times, short bursts of activity were usually associated with fear or anger, and our bodies still react to it in that way as anxiety and fight-or-flight emotions. Such short bursts are a body rhythm that people (excluding dedicated athletes and fitness enthusiasts) rarely engage in purposely. However, we can easily mimic the movement type with HIIT (high-intensity interval training) routines (explained later in this chapter).

These two basic rhythms are the same ones our ancestral bodies spent their days in foraging, hunting, or going about their prehistoric business, mostly related to food. While the danger-based short and fast rhythm was used only when necessary, nature gave it to us (and all creatures in the animal kingdom) as a tool in our survival kit, even though we spend most of our lives in the slow and even rhythm. In studying these two types, I realized that my body came to be what it is today *by moving most of the time.* All the systems and functions it relies on to keep me alive evolved into a lifestyle with movement as its heart. Thus, keeping myself moving made sense, as it could only benefit my health and my goals.

SERIOUS AEROBIC EXERCISE

The authors of *Younger Next Year* recommend doing serious (forty-five minutes a day) aerobic exercise at least four days a week at the following levels:

1. Long and even aerobic (60–65% of maximum heart rate or MHR)
2. Higher aerobic (70–85% of MHR), and
3. Maximum or anaerobic (90–100% of MHR)

Roughly 75 percent of our overall exercise time should hover in the lower aerobic range and 25 percent in the higher aerobic range. Maximum effort should be thrown in only occasionally, about once every week or two. (Note: In Part II, I have evolved this formula for my own practice. However, the *Younger Next Year* formula gave me a place to start and sustained me for years.)

THE VALUE OF STRENGTH TRAINING

Active movement isn't the only area that needs attention. Strength is equally important, especially given the weakness and atrophy that can occur in later life. *Younger Next Year*'s chapter on strength training involves gym equipment for standard routines of lifting and squatting. Again, this strength program provided a good place to start, but my basic yoga practice served me in more varied and subtle ways. Trying the gym routines, I found the range of motion this book recommended to be quite limited. Luckily, I hired a trainer who listened to my concerns. Together, we worked out a few routines that mimicked real-life coordinated movements. These became the basis for a whole new way of strength training that I explore in Part II.

In addition to *Younger Next Year*, I had read a few inspiring books on later life successes such as track athlete Olga Kotelko and yoga practitioner B.K.S. Iyengar, who remained fully functional and strong into their nineties. Their stories motivated me to include different forms of strength training in my practice. One's strength can be maintained and increased in a variety of ways, from using classic gym equipment to using my own body weight as resistance to doing yoga poses. I also grabbed opportunities to become stronger in daily living such as carrying groceries in two heavy bags instead of having them delivered or taking the stairs rather than using escalators. These became great ways to exercise in daily life as I became more aware of my body and appreciated its movement capabilities.

DAMAGE, STRESS, REPAIR, AND HEALING

Younger Next Year marked my first rudimentary exposure to the biochemistry of exercise and what eventually became a mantra for me. One key chapter stated that how we get stronger and rebuild and repair a muscle is by taxing it, actually damaging it slightly with our effort. This causes our friend the immune system to come to the rescue, remove the damaged tissue, and rebuild it *slightly stronger than before*. Nature has a way of minimizing the same kind of damage that occurs during movement by making it stronger. Imagine that!

This is an infinitely complex biochemical process involving inflammation, hormones, nutrients, and other dynamics. But this little morsel of knowledge resonated with something bigger inside me, that healing *stronger* is the result of a process involving stress and effort. Strength is caused by being challenged!

This process doesn't get learned; it's hardwired into my body. And it's part of the wonder of how I work. So I thought, "Surely if this process applies to muscles, it must apply to everything else inside me. I'll continue this kind of ongoing healing and repair into later life—the fountain of youth and an important factor in my longevity journey."

MOTIVATION, WILLPOWER, AND EFFORT

For the days I didn't feel like exercising, I devised a trade-off in my head, which was often enough to break through any motivational lapses. I simply told myself that for every hour I spend at the gym, I would get to live an extra day—an extra day to be with my daughters while they were growing up and an extra day to be alive. Talk about motivation! It worked virtually every time and still does on the off day when I'm under the spell of inertia. On the rare days it doesn't work, something else is going on; either I'm getting sick or something deep inside is brewing that I have to make room to digest.

Exercising regularly can be difficult. To begin with, willpower and effort are required. I bless that capacity in myself—that is, *knowing when something needs doing*. Even if I don't feel like it, I affirm that I'll be better off for doing it. In this sense, I am proactive, knowing that once I get going and can realize the benefits, exercising becomes easier. As my longtime yoga teacher said, "On days that you don't feel like practicing, just roll out the mat and sit on it, touch it, and do a quick pose or two." Preparing my mind and getting my blood flowing triggers my body to move. One simple movement like rolling out a gym mat invites spontaneity and breaks the inertia. Usually, a full session follows.

QUICK RESULTS

Results came quickly once I started a regular schedule. Within a few weeks, I was doing forty-five-minute sessions at the long, slow speeds as well as mixing in high speeds. Before long, I was able to sustain the high speeds longer and longer with less effort and breathing. This felt good. Ultimately, I could spend all my time in that high range while zoning out on the hundreds of songs loaded into my iPod.

In the gym, I used the stationary bike, stair climber, rowing machine, and treadmill for power walking. I mixed them up, depending on how I felt. Then I followed these sessions with stretching or yoga. On the days I didn't go to the gym, I did more intense yoga at home.

"Great!" I thought, once the routine was established. "This is what the experts recommend, and I'm doing it. Just keep this up, and I've got it made," I told myself. However, the stronger I got, the more I could see and deal with other areas that needed improvement. Although my progress was good, the long road to longevity still lay ahead.

Based on my experience, following *Younger Next Year* can be particularly good for people new to exercising and wanting to begin slowly. It provides background about the evolution of the human body and activities that keep us healthy and rejuvenated. Like the detox, taking a first step became more important than making sure it was precisely the right direction. Learning comes as much from experience as advice.

Following the book's recommendations gave me a positive first experience and a doable, regular routine. Plus, adding a heart monitor to my routines became a useful companion to understanding my cardiovascular health. Bringing exercise into my schedule every day has become an indispensable, non-negotiable habit that has added to my life—at that time and ever since.

COMING ALIVE

Increased movement and the bodily senses I've heightened have made me feel more alive. Medical evidence indicates this is the result of increased circulation and blood flow. In addition, I was in a better mood and life felt more hopeful and positive right after exercising. Thanks to detox and movement, I was living in my body more and my head less. "I'm headed in the right direction—the way life is supposed to be," I concluded.

In his book *The Body Keeps the Score*, psychiatrist Bessel van der Kolk states that movement and sensory experience provide a great way to reengage with our bodies—and to feel emotions related to old trauma and emotional scars buried inside. He also states that *not* living in our visceral bodies and feeling what they have to offer—merely *thinking* through life—allows us to not only avoid the pain associated with old scars but to deprive ourselves of the wonder and awe of experiencing life on a sensory level.

I now know that dealing with emotional issues is just as essential to the quality of life as diet and exercise, perhaps more. (More on this in chapters 14 and 21.)

A LESSON ON MOVEMENT IN AFRICA

Movement awakens all the senses. It also awakens old instincts no longer used for the same purposes. Here's an example.

Preceding and during the time I was discovering exercise, I was traveling regularly to East Africa, Tanzania, and Kenya. I went on several safaris and saw the animals and environment most people only view on BBC television or in *National Geographic*.

My most life-changing walking safari was in the Selous, one of the largest game reserves in Africa. The landscape was the typical dry scrub that makes up the Rufiji River region in the dry season. We walked in the wild upward of ten to fifteen miles a day for a week, mostly in the morning before the midday heat arrived. I've learned that this is roughly the same mileage our prehistoric ancestors covered daily in foraging or hunting for food.

There were six of us plus two guides. The guide in front carried a heavy-gauge loaded rifle that, if necessary, could bring down an elephant, rhino, or hippo. We slept outdoors in mosquito nets surrounded by nearby wildlife: lions, hippos, crocodiles, hyenas. And those were only the ones we could hear or see by the reflection of their eyes in our campfire or lanterns!

That environment was a far cry from tourist safaris experienced from the safety of a Land Rover and the shelter of a lodge. Once, a hippo charged us and our guide went down on one knee ready to shoot it but didn't have to; the hippo stopped. We all gingerly backed up, hearts racing. Another time, one of our cooks went to fetch water from a usually safe site next to Lake Tagalala. He was lunged at by a menacing crocodile, barely missing him. Luckily, his water pail was at the end of a long rope so he could escape. Another day, we came upon a group of Cape buffalo grazing. Luckily, we were downwind of them and made a hasty but very quiet retreat. The danger to us was real, palpable, and ever present.

Mostly, being on this safari felt surreal and magical—hearing, smelling, seeing, and touching the raw majesty of nature untamed by man. As much as I tried to feel "comfortable," I could not, yet I felt alive in ways I rarely do in our modern world. Likely our ancestors never felt too comfortable either; wariness and alertness were constants in their primal lives.

Most striking of all was how my sight, hearing, smell, and general instincts sharpened as never before. I developed reflexes that an unknown part of me orchestrated—*not* my conscious mind. Once, a scorpion dropped from a tree onto the shoulder of one of our guides right in front of me. Without thinking, I said, "Alex, don't move" and flicked it off him. While a scorpion bite might not have killed him, it would have been painful and could have ended our trip. I had never before done anything so instinctually.

This unknown ancestral memory reflex within me made me curious. "What else might awaken inside me?"

RECONNECTION TIME

After arriving home to London, I felt disoriented. City life felt dull and boring by comparison to being on the safari. Only my head, not my body, was engaged in city living; only exercise and movement reconnected me to that other world. I realized how different living had become from the time humans regularly engaged with nature symbiotically and energetically. I sensed my body needed to get reengaged in that way.

I began to not only appreciate the history and wonder of our human bodies but to be grateful for my body itself. Being active increased my sense of well-being immeasurably. For most of my life, I had not *liked* my body, based on what I looked like and how I felt about myself. Yet, it dawned on me that the vast, complex world of health inside me was a miracle that had nothing to do with self-judgment. *To the extent I made my body and health personal, I was missing the wonder of life itself.* I wanted to tap into *universal* health, a wonder shared by all living things.

That goal called for deeply appreciating the miracle of the human body, an exquisite combination of guts, chemistry, and biology. Our bodies were crafted over eons to become the latest version of *us*! Rather than criticizing it, I learned to appreciate my body for what it was intended for. I asked myself, "What has been my attitude toward my health and my body historically? And what beliefs spawned and sustained that attitude?" This was my first inkling that valuing oneself is a crucial part of health.

MY BODY, MY SELF

As a child, I was anything but athletic. I distinctly remember bouts of anguish over my inability to run and my lack of upper-body strength to do push-ups and pull-ups, all the rage among teenage boys. I was tall with a thin frame except for my hips and thighs, which were (and still are) big and powerful. I carried extra weight around my hips as chubbiness, resulting in a waistline bigger than my boyhood chest. My body was a source of shame and embarrassment to me, and I was mocked more than once about it.

When I became a teenager, my height and our high school's obsession with basketball brought me minor respectability playing a game in which height mattered. I could also throw and hit a baseball, so games of stickball in the parking lots of Newark became a regular pastime.

I had dreamt of having an attractive body, lean and muscular. As with most teenage boys, I compared my sadly lacking physique with my peers' and they with mine. I mistakenly thought having a good physique (like TV's fitness and nutrition guru Jack LaLanne) would make me more attractive to the popular girls in school. Longingly scouring comic book ads for weights showing muscle-bound guys, I fantasized about the number of girls I'd attract if I only had those pecs. Yet, I never did anything except daydream.

JOBS BUILT MY STRENGTH

Thankfully, as I got older, my ability to take on tough physical jobs gave me self-respect toward my body. I worked my way through college at various hard labor jobs: loading and unloading trucks and railroad cars; repairing railroad tracks and bunkers in a dynamite and gunpowder factory; laying, cutting, and carrying wall-to-wall carpet; doing carpentry and woodworking; carrying supplies at a construction site; landscaping; and even taking a summer job on a sanitation truck. (That was the only job I ever quit; I just couldn't take that one.) Doing these jobs, I didn't talk back and could endure many hours, including overtime. People liked my responsible efficiency, and I was good at the work.

After college, I built houses as a carpenter. Given that I was the new guy, the first six months mostly called for carrying lumber around. I also spent my days hammering nails, pushing, pulling, lifting, climbing ladders, balancing, kneeling, crouching, and bending. Through all this movement, I eventually acquired the lean muscles I longed for—and became proud of my body. That, combined with my brain, helped me earn a living and made me strong.

BECOMING SEDENTARY

By my late twenties, though, all that had changed. I had begun my lifelong career in the printing business—first as a salesman for, and later an owner of, the printing company mentioned earlier. I sorely missed the way my body felt and the strength I had in those blue-collar days. My lower back bothered me, so I began aerobic exercises after reading Ken Cooper's *The Aerobics Way*. I also saw chiropractors and back doctors for my aching back.

Walking and biking the streets of New York City, either to or from work or in Central Park on weekends, supplemented my irregular visits to a gym. I had always loved fast walking, although running was not my forte because it tired me out faster than any other exercise. I'd be huffing and puffing before I knew it.

To my relief, I took up swimming around age forty. I swam every day for stress relief as well as physical fitness. Eventually, I joined a local Masters team and even participated in low-level meets among my peers. Intense swimming kept off the weight I would have gained from endless dining and drinking entertainment. Along with doing yoga to help my back, that's how I spent the next fifteen to twenty years of my physical fitness life.

At the time, I wasn't aware of the deeper benefits I was giving myself by my once-a-day exercise routine. Specifically, I was providing my brain and organs with the benefits of increased circulation. Still, exercise was about looking good, feeling good, and allowing me to eat and drink whatever I wanted. The newer dimensions of the somatic reconnection with my emotions only came once I realized the instinctual symbiosis of movement and health.

SYMBIOTIC HEALTH

The health of our vital organs and brain are as important for longevity as healthy legs, abdominals, and biceps. To have a well-functioning body, no area should be neglected; every part of the body relies on and supports every other. All the parts are exquisitely interconnected. Aerobics keeps the blood moving and heart strong. Combined with the subtle and far-reaching aspects of a practice like yoga, every body part is reached. Yet the importance of movement is more than just physical; *it's a kind of energy that affirms life*. The physical organism that is *me* is no less me than my brain or soul or mind. Indeed, my ability to think comes from the blood and guts inside me. I regard this as a masterpiece of natural engineering. Nature is supremely efficient.

NEW WHEELS SPINNING

In my fifties and early sixties, new wheels were spinning. A vast hidden world inside me, the one sparked while on the train ride, began to exert a bigger pull, providing a launching point for the next big phase of my journey, perhaps the most critical. Attitude, belief, and self-awareness have all become integral to leading a long, healthy life. In a conventional medical sense, we usually don't associate these aspects with health or longevity. Yet when I raise the point about this integration in conversation, most people sense the link between the two.

Chapters 5, 6, and 7 address subtle aspects of the next part of my journey, describing how this truth was revealed and how it ultimately changed everything.

5

Profound Change Begins

*"Tell me, what is it you plan to do with
your one wild and precious life?"*
—MARY OLIVER

My main focus revolved around spending time with and providing for my family, smoothing out a few rough edges along the way. One of my businesses was having problems, while another was doing well. The third one never got off the ground. I had also staged a few theatrical productions with mixed commercial success (the norm in that highly risky field). But no matter how hard I tried, it didn't look like I'd be back in the high life of fame and fortune anytime soon. Life did me a favor on that score. *That's not where I was meant to be looking for answers.*

As I experimented with diet and exercise, everything I read showed a clear correlation among health, movement, and what to eat and avoid. Most of what I was practicing was science-based—medically "proven" advice from books and online sources. But other less tangible, more subtle factors affect longevity that interested me as well: lifestyle, social and family life, heritage and genes, purpose and meaning, and inner life and beliefs.

SUBTLE FACTORS OF HEALTH

Many questions arose for me around these new factors:

- How did lifestyle affect my health?
- How happy and content was I with my life?
- Did I feel positive about the future?
- Did I feel my life had meaning?
- What was my attitude toward getting older and entering this new phase of life? Was it seen as a slow decline or a new, vital chapter?
- Did how I live and who I spent my time with affect my health?
- What about my genes and my past?
- What about my parents' view of a life they never got to experience?
- How did this all combine inside to bring about the best results?
- How important was all this in helping me live longer and better?
- Would just copying someone else's healthy lifestyle automatically give me one?
- Was my work and how I spent my time important to my health?

Clearly, I had many more questions than answers. I'd always headed toward books to find answers—and this time was no exception. I continued my reading on any topic even vaguely related. Among the subjects of my eclectic collection of books on "the project" (as I called it) were evolution, writing, psychology, modern and alternative medicine, longevity and aging studies, healthy older populations, Zen Buddhism, philosophy, and meaning.

THE MIRACLE OF CHANGE

As important as digesting all this material, though, I had a powerful sense of *new inner resources* stirring inside. Having been awakened, the forces of change within me gained momentum, slowly evolving into a trusted and guiding inner power. I believe I was experiencing the miracle of change, not by choice but by inspiration.

When a heartfelt yearning to know is tapped, it serves to heal us. Our yearning moves us in new directions while gaining support from a buried, infinitely resourceful part of ourselves. That part of us that is primal and healthy, that seeks wholeness and seamlessness is a common heritage.

I realized how this research was meant to deepen and expand the work I'd begun on the train. Physical health was a mystery I had taken for granted most of my life, yet hitting my sixties changed all that. But what if the truth was the other way around? *What if how I felt about myself and my life determined my physical health?*

Currents of truth run deep through our subconscious minds without us even knowing. Self-love, appreciation, worthiness, and their opposites—self-hate and scorn—are central players on this battlefield. They often determine how grateful and passionate we feel about life *and* how much we want (or deserve) to be healthy to enjoy it. Thinking this way turned everything about health and longevity on its head for me. *It affected the core sense of who I am.* How did all these ideas come together and stay with me? My breakthrough happened by tackling my worst health habit.

BOOZE AND MY RELATIONSHIP WITH IT

If I pointed to one issue of concern standing in the way of achieving my health and longevity goals, it was drinking alcohol. While eating well and exercising might minimize the damage drinking alcohol caused, they alone would not solve the unsolvable, no matter how hard I tried to rationalize it. The research was clear: alcohol's negative effect on my body as I aged would become even more pronounced if I continued to drink.

My norm was drinking a big cocktail (or two)—either gin or scotch—before dinner. That was followed with at least a half bottle—sometimes a whole bottle—of wine during dinner. Whether cocktails or dinner parties, theater outings, airplanes and lounges, or socializing with clients and employees, drinking alcohol accompanied every event—a constant companion. No matter how much I tried to stop at one or two or even three, I couldn't.

While I could hold alcohol well and only sometimes become sloppy or drunk, I didn't doubt that the amount I was drinking would shorten my life—and lead to a chronic condition that would impair my later years.

I began drinking as a teenager of seventeen, sneaking beers with the boys or stealing liquor from our parents' cupboards. I was amazed how much courage I felt under its influence, not only eliminating my shyness but giving me extra courage to be bold. Alcohol and I were the perfect match, sustaining each other as best friends and my go-to resource in times of trouble. My early college life was filled with beer at dorm and fraternity parties. Rutgers, the university I attended, allowed drinking on campus. When I joined a fraternity, guess who was in charge of the kegs of beer? Me! Once I had a drink, everything felt okay inside. Beer loosened me up, gave me courage, made dancing and approaching girls easier, turned any blues into silliness, and generally numbed my practical, responsible, and quiet side. I liked myself better and felt more social under the influence.

When I was twenty-two and after my mother's funeral, I knocked back a few brandies put out for guests. The sweet numbness felt like heaven after the tears I had shed shoveling the first clods of earth on her coffin. Over time, social drinking became a necessary accompaniment to evening activities, social or otherwise. If I knew there'd be no alcohol where I was going, I'd make sure to have some beforehand.

Messages from My Daughter

As I've said, I was "lucky" I could hold alcohol well and not get "drunk"—only happy and loose—to the point that most people would be surprised to learn alcohol was a problem for me. This became part of my rationalizing. But inside, I knew I drank too much despite secretly trying to cut down or quit for years.

One day, I brought home a book called *The Easy Way to Stop Drinking*. My then one-year-old newly walking daughter Jessica would repeatedly pick out that book from the middle of a stack and bring it to me. It became a game between us, but it sent me an insistent message. "Look, Daddy," she seemed to be saying, "read *this* book."

Admittedly, my mornings after drinking were foggy, which I did not like. Mornings had always been my favorite time of the day; it was when my daughters and I spent much of our time together. And my wife often said she liked me hung over because I was more relaxed and fun, even though I felt miserable.

Buying Acceptance

My affluent lifestyle and the trappings of two successful careers were as addictive as the alcohol. Together, they conveyed the image

I wanted to convey—that I was worldly, successful, generous, admirable, and low-key yet could be stern when necessary. That image of myself underlay much of my drive—always fueled by alcohol. I had wine cellars or giant wine coolers for proper storage in my New York and London homes. I was proud of owning, serving, ordering, and giving as gifts the finest wines on the planet.

Cost was rarely an object, especially when paid for by lavish entertainment expense accounts. I always picked up the check, seeing it in my role as supporter and provider. As generous as others thought I was, it was my way of secretly feeling superior or, at least, adequate. It was also my way of buying acceptance because, privately, I thought people might not like me otherwise. Yet, as I eventually learned, the source of those private thoughts was *me not liking myself.*

False Security

When I had previously tried to curtail my drinking, I came up against losing all that false security. I was also up against becoming as shy, quiet, and withdrawn as I'd been in my youth. I felt desperate to avoid that, knowing it would leave me open to a wall of self-criticism. I had no idea how big that wall was at the time.

Yet something in me said, "This is the only way forward, come what may." I remember what Doctor One said about my drinking: "I thought you said you would do *anything* to stick around for your children." That one sentence haunted me. Along with all the research that pointed to the ill effects and increased risks of alcohol misuse, I realized no possible compromise was available; *I simply had to face head-on whatever might lay before me.* Even if it meant only one extra year of healthy life, it would be worth the effort.

If this seems overly dramatic, I assure you that my fear of losing alcohol was up there among the scariest moments of my life—as big turning points are.

WHEN I STOPPED

So, one morning I just stopped, cold turkey, after the previous night's cocktail party in which I had overindulged. Whatever powers cause us to see new options and change our ways worked their wonder on me. I knew from my detox experience that if I could get through the first few weeks and start experiencing the positive side of quitting, stopping would become much easier—and it did.

My physical and mental health have benefitted greatly from quitting drinking. Yet it also has changed me in the way I'd feared—making me shyer and less lively in social situations. No longer was I the one who stayed out dancing until all hours of the night. This shift felt awkward and difficult, especially at first. I was inclined to sit back and be thoughtful, introspective, and afraid of engaging with others, even boring. Imagine! I was condemning myself for not being the life of the party and judging myself unfairly in the process.

Still, my health, longevity, and promises I made to my children and myself were singularly more important than drinking. I never regretted initiating this change and am immensely grateful for doing so. It forced me to recognize the part of me I was so desperately trying to cover up. I realized my quiet side was the part I'd secretly relied on to make big decisions. It was more instinctual, heartfelt, genuine, and other worldly than my public business personality. It felt as though that aspect sprang from an unknown yet highly trusted part of me, like the voice of conscience—the same voice I had heard that day on the train ride.

PROTECTING MY IMAGE

The part of me I had kept out front was the worldly man, successful and accomplished, who lived internationally and moved through different geo-socio-religious and economic strata with ease and grace. My image of being understanding, gracious, and charming was also brittle, as I could be harsh, angry, and demanding at the same time. For years, I had so little awareness of the depths of my being and how everything inside works that I needed the false confidence of this brusque image to function. My strengths and weaknesses—what mattered and what I really needed—had been hidden from me. I had become blind to what would be my present life, acknowledging and accepting who I really am. My awareness of *real power* and knowing the *real me* started when I stopped drinking. I no longer had a place to hide.

Simply put, I stopped pushing my *real self* into the background, but how could I make sure it became a big part of my life? At first, I didn't know; I only knew at cocktail parties and other social situations, I felt extremely awkward without drinking. Still, I forced myself to confront those feelings as honestly as I could. It was hard. I felt like I was firing on two cylinders instead of eight. I shunned and disparaged that awkward side of me for a long time, but eventually, I did manage the change.

I allowed myself the time, patience, and benevolence to tolerate the new tension, accepting it as part of a bigger process. I watched and listened for answers while letting life happen. During this time, I found myself drawn to different types of people, which told me this new presence had been with me—and invisible—all my life. As I opened my world, I realized that certain people I had shunned and labeled "plain, not cool" were more substantial human beings than the "popular" ones I had wanted to be with.

ABRUPT CHANGE IN DIRECTION

Once I decided to stop drinking, my abrupt change in direction became dogged and determined in the face of mixed reactions from friends and family. In most cases, they weren't too supportive, and some were downright disapproving. Although this hurt me, they did not sway my determination. What was tolerating their disapproval compared to living longer and staying healthy? If I hadn't been so single-minded and able to withstand their kidding ("c'mon, just one drink won't hurt you"), I might have lapsed. At first, I had no way of knowing my resolve touched something in *their* lives that frightened them. I just gritted my teeth to get through.

Truth be told, part of me no longer wanted to live in that conventional, gossipy world, so *no more drinking* marked my first concrete step out of it. In *The War of Art*, Steven Pressfield had choice words about the resistance to change from so-called loving friends and family. He wrote: "Often couples or close friends, even entire families, will enter into tacit compacts whereby each individual pledges (unconsciously) to remain mired in the same slough in which he or she and all her cronies have become so comfortable. The highest treason a crab can commit is to make a leap for the rim of the bucket."[1]

Yes, I wanted out of that bucket despite the disparagement. Being afraid of rejection is typically the reason people don't act, yet I can assure you, the payoff of positive inner change has outweighed any rejection. *And* I found people who were supportive, those who appreciated me even more due to my quiet behavior.

HEALTH EFFECTS AND PSYCHOTHERAPY

The health effects of stopping drinking were profound. I had more energy, better sleep, much improved digestion—and these were only the first immediately obvious changes. I had temporarily felt the same benefits during the detox. Would they become permanent? I hoped so.

In addition, I knew I'd stopped giving my immune system and liver a vast load of unnecessary work. Now they could focus on what they were intended to do: keep my insides clean and protect me from actual pathogens (not the poisons I was pumping into myself every night by the low-level bottleful). The period that followed ushered in expansive changes. First, I started psychotherapy again to nurse the self-discovery process I'd begun. At this time, I needed the support of a professional to help guide me and stand firmly in my corner. My wife's disapproval with my changes was growing louder, but so was my inner rallying cry to defend my new lifestyle.

The truth be told, my wife and I started having issues before my decision to quit, but that step greatly increased the friction between us. I wanted to have a life partner who supported and respected my choices, especially those in the best interest of our family and my role in it. Yet, my increasingly unconventional views were not to her liking, even after I explained how and why I was doing them. Her friends did not embrace them either, and when I stopped drinking, the disapproval deepened.

My worst fear? That we would separate, which would strongly affect not only our marriage but our children. For the first time in a long while, I started to pray. I asked to be shown the way forward and admitted I needed a different kind of help. This was also the first time I enlisted the forces of the universe—all the things that could affect me, inside and outside, that are beyond my immediate control. I begged that these universal forces show me the way. In the long run, they played a bigger role in my belief system than I could ever foresee.

At the same time, I had a vastly increased amount of free time since I no longer spent every night getting plastered and every morning recovering. I could have more quality time with my daughters and with my work. But it wasn't *business* work I turned to. Researching health issues, writing, doing self-analysis, journaling, and deeply pondering became my preferred way to spend this golden, sacred time. My health-related activities were taking on a deeper spiritual quality, especially my yoga practice. My yoga teacher had hinted about its spiritual side, and although I recognized it intellectually, I rarely felt it viscerally—until now.

NEED TO TACKLE SOURCES OF HABITS

In *The Story of the Human Body*, Dr. Daniel Lieberman makes the case that many of our modern-day maladies result from the mismatch between our bodies and the activities we've evolved toward in modern living. He points to sitting in chairs, consuming excessive amounts of sugar, and wearing constrictive shoes as examples of harmful habits.

Yet he stops short of asking the deeper questions: Why do we continue to harm ourselves in ways like these? Why is it simply not enough *knowing* that something is unhealthy for us to change our behavior? Why doesn't the purely rational side of our brain have the strength to effect actual change?

I realized I couldn't truly change inside through willpower. I couldn't force myself to shift habits that no longer supported me.

Rather, the *source* of those habits needed to be tackled and understood. And those sources, I found out, lay in the emotional connections inside me.

Drinking allowed me to suppress the symptoms of my inner struggle, but *real* healing involved discomfort, friction, and most of all, effort and faith. It also involved emotional healing, which includes self-understanding and self-appreciation beyond any physical symptoms. And while it was *not* the last time I ever touched a drink (today, I occasionally drink limited amounts), for seven or eight years after I decided to quit for good, I didn't touch a drop of alcohol. This discovery-filled break from alcohol formed the basis of the life I live today.

6

The World Within

"I believe that psychogenic physical disorders (that is, disorders induced by emotions) develop because of undesirable or frightening repressed feelings."
—DR. JOHN SARNO

The more I trusted my fledgling inner health compass to guide me, the more I was drawn to the world inside. I clearly needed to explore it in depth, as it directly affected my health and longevity. My awakening on the train ride had led me to develop healthy habits as the focus for my physical body's health. Now, a more comprehensive picture of what made me tick was starting to dawn.

All this led to a more expansive landscape: *health and quality of life depend on more than diet and exercise.* While they counted for a lot, the root causes and cures of disease were only partially addressed by changing unhealthy habits. *Why* did people get sick in the first place, not just *how*?

MY BACK: A PSYCHOPHYSICAL HISTORY

I had an inkling of a mind-body connection years ago. As a young man during college and afterward, I worked a variety of hard, hands-on, blue-collar jobs. In my twenties, I got occasional lower back spasms, often severely incapacitating. They seemed to strike at random, came out of nowhere, and couldn't be tied to any specific activity. A range of orthopedists, chiropractors, and osteopaths advocated a combination of rest, spinal adjustments, massage, pain relievers, anti-inflammatories, and anything else to relax the affected muscles.

Sometimes rest worked; other times it did not. Activity usually made me feel better, but sometimes it didn't. Muscle relaxers and alcohol would help occasionally or at least numb the pain enough to give me that impression. I even saw the same doctor that President Kennedy had used for his bad back, Hans Kraus, who had developed a radical theory of pressure points and ice treatment. Unfortunately, this approach didn't work on me.

THE WORK OF DR. JOHN SARNO

At some point in looking for effective treatments, I ran across the work of Dr. John Sarno, a doctor at NYU Medical Center Institute of Rehabilitative Medicine. He had written several books about what he called tension myositis syndrome (TMS) as being not only the cause of most back pain but a host of other health issues.

Dr. Sarno's theory is this: Anxiety and subconscious inner conflict, unexpressed emotions, and particularly anger can create a temporary lessening of blood flow to muscles, causing them to weaken and spasm. He suggests that when your back goes out, you want to recall what you were thinking and feeling at that moment. The pain means something has been triggered in your subconscious, causing the TMS and subsequent attack.

This was far-out stuff in the 1970s and '80s. Dr. Sarno himself, despite helping huge numbers of people who praised him in reviews, was never accepted by the medical community as offering a valid, provable diagnosis and treatment. Nonetheless, I did acknowledge that a partial cause for my bad back might be psychological or psychophysical. The more I entertained the notion and practiced his technique, the more it brought me relief and a speedier recovery.

Why are backs the area of the body where TMS attacks? It's likely due to the amount of time we spend seated. Sitting can weaken our lower backs and hips to such an extent that they become weak and vulnerable. Blood flow is already restricted, and the TMS exacerbates this condition. As Dr. Sarno writes, because back problems have become so commonplace, they've also become an accepted and shared form of disability. As a result, social and belief factors are at work as well.

At a certain point in my early forties, I started doing hatha yoga, which helped strengthen my back, hips, and legs enough to better integrate how my body moved. My back spasms stopped. If I have a rare incident, I can usually release the discomfort with breathing and yoga twists. And knowing from Dr. Sarno's work that the spasm isn't entirely physical makes the muscle easier to release.

THE POWER OF BELIEF ON THE BODY

The world of mind/body disorders doesn't stop with bad backs or tense muscles. The more I read, the more it became apparent that what people believe affects their health—both positively and negatively—including the actual condition of their bodies. Given that our physical biology serves as the evolutionary foundation of our minds and emotions, the intimate connection between the two became obvious to me.

Yet, surprisingly, this connection hasn't been widely accepted in modern medicine. Placebo studies[1] are often overlooked and usually downplayed as drug companies rush their products to market. Yet the evidentiary results of drug studies show that placebos (giving patients who are ill fake copies of a drug) can be as effective as the actual drug. In many cases, placebos are even more effective than drugs, which results in a "failed" study—that is, not enough positive results to bring the drug to market. Depending on the drug and the condition, placebos work in 20 to 70 percent of patients—results based purely on belief. In one novel BBC/Oxford University study, *all* the participants were unknowingly given placebos for severe back pain, yet half of them still got better! The participants stimulate healing or alleviation of pain by their belief. So, if we can tap into the body's ability to heal itself through our beliefs, then the opposite must be true as well: *People can become ill from the beliefs they hold.* (See bibliography for studies and resources.)

SICK BODY OR SICK SOUL?

Soon after I began experimenting with my health, I had a conversation with my mother-in-law about my search for health and longevity. While she was too diplomatic to disagree, I could tell she was wary of my findings and disagreed with my outlook. I told her I was determined to live my later years with as much activity and energy as I could. Her response: "I'm not sure the price of getting old, losing your looks, and becoming frail and sick are worth the extra years." She was in her midsixties at the time.

Her eldest brother, her large family's patriarch, had recently died of brain cancer. She spoke often of how deeply she was affected by his passing. Sadly, less than four years later, she also passed away before her seventieth birthday. A melanoma had been diagnosed and removed about fifteen years earlier but had asymptomatically metastasized in various organs of her body. By the time this became apparent, the cancer was already stage IV.

Her roller coaster battle with the disease was marked by a swift decline and then a yearlong reprieve due to a newly approved drug that targeted specific cancers and gene types. During it all, I couldn't get our earlier conversation out of my head, although I kept it to myself. *Was there something about her attitude toward how she viewed herself and the onset of her later years that contributed to this rapid escalation?*

Granted, she was a lifelong smoker, sparking obvious finger pointing. Some people even said she could be demanding and that her underlying temper could have fueled her disease. The frenzy of people who gave advice and shared their version of causes seemed endless. The ones who distracted her and made her laugh helped the most. Yet over the course of her sickness, she slowed down and became deeply appreciative of every day. Her mornings where she lived in East Africa were filled with sunshine and birds singing, which she listened to in a state of calm, peace, and grace. This was how I will remember her.

Through this sad experience, I learned that appreciating and acknowledging the wonder of being alive—and the power it holds—might be a dominant factor in supporting health and longevity. It's possible that *not liking myself* could have an outsized effect on the quality of my health. I had already seen how underground emotions caused my unhealthy habit of drinking. At this point, the synergy between the two realms was plainly evident.

PERSONAL RESONANCE

This synergistic connection resonated deeply within. Then one day it dawned on me. As much as I was working on promoting health and delaying death, I had never fully processed the early deaths of my own parents. My father died at age forty-seven and my mother at fifty-five, both from cancer. My mother-in-law's passing brought my hidden emotions to the surface and made me realize I had suppressed my early experience with death in favor of pursuing success and achievement. Now, in my quest for continued health and longevity, my emotional memory began to have an immense effect.

My father's death is more mysterious to me than my mother's. I was only seven when he died. I remember him as happy and responsible, someone I played with and laughed with a lot. His untimely death left a big hole in my life.

I was twenty-two when my mother died. I experienced how deeply unhappy and volatile she was for the fifteen years after my father died, and I took the brunt of these emotions. She had been a lifelong two-pack-a-day smoker, which didn't help anything. Her self-defined sentence of punishment played a big role in her sickness along with the physical factors. Neither of my parents had experienced anything like the kind of healthy later life I was working toward and hoping for.

As I let these emotions and memories process in their own rhythm, it dawned on me that the quality and perhaps the length of my later life might be affected by my own happiness—how I felt about myself and how I dealt with my time. From these examples as well as others from experience and literature (like *The Death of Ivan Ilyich* by Leo Tolstoy), feelings and beliefs about life, especially mine, became intricately tied to the physical practice I had initiated.

ASKING GUT QUESTIONS

How do emotions and beliefs factor into our health? Does the body get sick or the soul?

I had never asked myself these questions. As much as the medical community doesn't want to entertain a mind-body link, most people know in their guts that one exists. Science writer Jo Marchant's *CURE* has explored the terrain of placebos, biology, and belief. To her surprise, she found the connections too numerous to be discounted, that they deserve a place in modern medical diagnosis. Other scientists and doctors such as Dr. John Sarno and Dr. Mark Hyman who believe in mind-body connections have tried to map out how the communication happens. Their work on the vagus nerve (the cranial nerve that interfaces with the parasympathetic control of the heart, lungs, and digestive tract) and other pathways is encouraging. In my opinion, it represents the frontier of a field in which there's much to learn.

I've lived many examples of the interrelationship between body and psyche. They range from the effects of my bad back to digestion issues exacerbated by stress to energy in abundance when I felt good versus low energy during episodes of self-criticism to low immune function and illness when under stress. Instinctually, I knew my body was capable of miraculous and mysterious inner communication. This integrated connection operating on many levels could not be overlooked. It had to play a big part in my mission to create a healthy life in my later years.

7

Serendipity
Letting Life Guide Me

"The fact that highly implausible events, for which no cause can be determined within the framework of known natural law, occur with implausible frequency has come to be known as the principle of synchronicity."
—M. SCOTT PECK, *The Road Less Traveled*

As an active and involved dad, my daughters have always been my priority. My life revolved around them, whether it was school-related or weekend activities. My older daughter who had started nursery and then kindergarten was noticing I was older than other fathers, despite my keeping up with or exceeding them energy wise. Yet she and her sister also knew I was around more than the other dads at home and at school. I had devoted the rest of my time to financially supporting the family and, increasingly, to my health research and practice. (See the bibliography for a myriad of books I have studied through this journey.)

DIFFICULT TERRAIN

During this time of intense learning, the more I plunged into the research, the more fascinated I became as I incorporated the practices

I was developing. As far as having support for it, though, the terrain was difficult. I could only count on the few friends who'd been there for me when I stopped drinking. Also, beyond my health, I was often on shaky ground—feeling anxious and uncomfortable. My new physical strength didn't translate into mental ease. The further I diverged from my old ways, the more resistance I perceived inside. And as much as I believed I was on to something, explaining what I was doing to others wasn't easy. Why? Partly because my journey was all new to me. And partly because people rarely shared the same interest or saw their lives in the same way I was experiencing mine.

Some of this could be attributed to age and stage of life. Most of the people I knew were younger than me and in the thrall of their careers and young families. Ambition, status, image, and current circumstances are powerful forces that can limit one's options and viewpoints. Clinging to old ways formed the basis of my own anxiety and resistance. I shouldn't have been surprised by the resistance of others. Somehow, though, I had expected them to be as enthralled with my experience as I was. Not so.

I have since learned that my journey is best served by continuing this work with or without approval from others. The only validation I needed resides inside me. But back then, I wasn't strong enough to acknowledge and accept this truth or hear the new voice inside me as clearly as I can now.

HEED THE SIGNS

Life has a way of showing us signs, and several showed up around the time my daughters were young. These seemed to come at just the right moment.

The first sign was being introduced to John Donovan by a mutual friend, Marty Keller. John was leading a weekly discussion and therapy group that Marty participated in. In this supportive group environment, people discussed their problems out loud while working to uncover roads to solve them.

John is a respected, highly effective, yet unconventional counselor and substance abuse recovery expert. He calls himself a "recovered redneck" and a "recovery junkie." He's developed ways of allowing people he works with to realize their inner power and make changes. John feels especially adamant about one thing: *All the good wishes and benevolence in the world won't change people until they feel their own suffering and resolve to change themselves.*

In addition to being a recovered alcoholic, John had a health experience that dovetailed directly with the work I was doing. He recovered from prostate cancer but had refused his doctor's recommended medical treatment of surgery and/or radiation. Instead, he went to a medical nutritionist and changed his diet from one of comfort food to healthy, fresh foods. He also eliminated anything processed or sweet. John lost over thirty pounds and gave his immune system the much-needed strength to fight the cancer.

Because he believed in a self-created emotional component to physical disease, John did a deep therapeutic intervention on himself to uncover whether his inner emotional status was contributing to his cancer. One part stuck—that cancer is activated by long-held resentment, anger, or deep hurt that hasn't been allowed to heal. The other part seems obvious—that the prostate is a male organ. He sensed that the two together contributed to resenting the responsibilities of being a man, specifically always having to be strong, hard, tough, proud, and infallible as opposed to letting his softer, more sensitive, emotional side be heard. Many men, including John and me, have gotten trapped into playing a role that limits other avenues of growth.

His healing work involved a seismic confrontation with events from his past, which resulted in his small prostate tumor disappearing and his PSA returning to low levels. Talking with John was like hearing the ideas I was working on being played back in real time.

LETTING GO

John and I discussed my own drinking and recovery. From him, I learned about a vast community of people who went through (or are going through) what I had, sparking an inner history of what alcohol meant for them. While I hadn't attended Alcoholics Anonymous to help me stop, my journey was much the same as those who had. Uncovering what *caused* me to drink heavily helped me realize how much my hidden inner life was driving who I was and how I lived.

There was also the letting go aspect, trusting in something bigger than the world I can control. Everyone has a version of this, whether that something is deep inside them or from the outside. Yet those vast forces are more mysteriously powerful than most are willing to admit. Then I saw it! *Whatever force helped me realize the state of my life on the train was the same guide who gave me the insight and strength to stop drinking and begin my longevity work.*

THE SECOND SIGN

On a flight back from New York with my family, due to an airline mistake, I sat with my daughters in economy while my wife sat in premium economy one cabin up. I was fuming as we sat down in our two cramped seats with my almost-one-year-old daughter on my lap in the center seat of three. She was squirming and being very vocal. My almost-four-year-old daughter sat in the aisle seat next to me. The man who sat quietly and peacefully next to me at the window offered to help. I apologized for the fuss.

As the long flight got going, I calmed down and we started talking. His name was Michael Suarez, an American and English professor at Oxford University and a Jesuit priest. Today, he heads the Rare Books School at the University of Virginia where he is a professor. Once I got going, I told him the entire story of my previous few years—the moment on the train, the deep feeling of mortality, my daughters, the work, the research, the practice—all of it. He completely understood what I was saying without my explaining further and without asking a single question. He deemed my mission worthwhile—rare in today's world—and said I should keep pursuing it.

We talked the entire flight, interrupted only by my daughters, on subjects ranging from health to Dante's *Divine Comedy*. He commented that having a meaning in life was something most people don't even know they're missing and said I was lucky to have found a path toward purpose. He also pointed me to the poet and essayist Mary Oliver, saying I'd find kinship with my mission in her writing. In particular, he cited her essay "Of Power and Time" from the collection *Blue Pastures*. Its last line still hangs over my desk:

> *"The most regretful people on earth are those who felt the call to creative work, who felt their own creative power restive and uprising, and who gave it neither power nor time."*[1]
>
> —MARY OLIVER

Talk about a mantra for life and a remedy for regret!

I came off that flight feeling the universe had granted me a wish and given me strength, light, and direction. The encounter made me realize there *were* people who understood and appreciated what I was doing. Even more, Michael showed me that my journey echoed the same universal search that artists, philosophers, teachers, and religious figures had undertaken through the ages.

It comes up differently in each one of us, but ultimately we are striving for something more expansive than ourselves—an unlived life, a deeper awareness, a longing to know more. It felt good to have been heard and appreciated by Michael—a sign that *I wasn't alone in this after all!* Whatever forces were guiding me were getting stronger, or I was allowing them to. That meant my instinct of looking for clues about health and longevity outside the norm weren't far-fetched at all.

LEARNING FROM EVOLUTION

I was committed to understanding how my body functioned and what I could do to keep myself healthy. To accomplish this, I had a burning desire to learn how the organism I know as "me" had come to be through eons of prehistoric history.

I could work on the "software" aspect of my commitment by studying my lifestyle, my past, and my inner life, but knowing the "hardware" aspect was another matter. Nature had done all that work before I was born by crafting and honing the miraculous organism that I am (and we all are). Learning about the dynamics of evolution would serve me in my quest for health and longevity. I couldn't stop asking, "How did I get here and why?"

In our modern world of convenience, comfort, and readily available food, we can forget the forces that shaped our bodies. Yes, we were built to survive and overcome challenges, but this "great guide" of evolution is more than survival of the fittest. Our bodies and minds and whatever keeps them healthy all come from eons of generations of evolution. We humans owe those generations a debt of gratitude for our existence. Their struggles led to the dawning of consciousness and our eventual entry into modern life. I believe that the more I could harmonize with those primitive qualities plus the activities and nutrients that shaped the evolutionary process, the healthier I would become.

My interest in evolution dovetailed with my thoughts about God, what guides the universe, and why and how we continue to exist. I couldn't get enough of this exposure to the natural world before humans became conscious or self-aware—about 50,000 to 100,000 years ago, a millisecond in evolutionary time.

DEVELOPMENT OF CONSCIOUSNESS

Consciousness—the awareness that separates humans from other forms of life—sprang from and still exists due to visceral biology. Its development was ultimately a biological process, yet based on my reading, no one has explained the wonder of an abstract thought or the biochemistry of neurons and brain impulses. The universe had been doing well without this newly developed ability, it seemed.

But once human consciousness happened, we forever left the land of "what is" and encountered life as a mixture of "what is, what could be, and what should be." Don't get me wrong; 90 percent of us still operate under the radar on ancient rhythms. But since becoming conscious, our waking lives became a composite of emotion and imagination, which gave us power over the world around us. As Joseph Campbell documents in his many works, ever since that time, humans have been trying to come to grips with the source of our existence and our abilities. This puzzle has taken on many iterations but is one we haven't come close to solving.

I have come to understand that my body and psyche were formed by evolution over millions of years. The vast bulk of this time, 95 percent or more, my ancestors roamed the East African plains in an environment and conditions that produced the body I have. My experiences in Africa provided a testament to my own body's knowledge and memory of this. Africa is where my ancestors learned to stand, walk on two legs, and nourish themselves on available food. Instinctively, my body feels most attuned to their movements and nutrition and experiences. By knowing my ancestors thrived under those conditions, being in tune with their lifestyles would serve me well.

Yet one aspect of my evolutionary biology is more subtle. Living in my somatic body required *experiencing* the emotional realities of life as opposed to *thinking* my way through them. These emotions formed a deeper basis for many aspects of my life than I realized.

Living in the emotional world of problems—feeling them and sensing how to tackle them—was occurring for me frequently. The experience wasn't always pleasant, yet it usually ended up being where solutions and resolutions were found. I was learning that my visceral attraction to this world—in both biological and emotional terms—was being guided by an even larger healing power than I'd ever been aware of before.

8

Healing a Family Disaster

"I thought I'd die, but I didn't."
—PEGGY LEE, "IS THAT ALL THERE IS?"

For much of my life, my singular desire was to have a family—one I didn't have except for the precious few years before my father died. The dysfunction that ensued, his absence, and my mother's all-consuming grief had erased my emotional memory of family. It was replaced by the unharmonious unit that my mother and I formed. Neither of our needs were being met during the years we spent together. I deeply longed to be part of a family environment that could change that dynamic.

And now I had one, complete with my own children to bring up differently than I had been raised. I'd give them as much love as I could; I'd nourish them and heal myself at the same time. Yet things between my wife and me had soured, not as "made for each other" rosy as they once were. Our relationship became especially hard after my financial troubles and my turn toward health and inner life explorations.

MARRIAGE AS BASE CAMP

In *The Road Less Traveled*, M. Scott Peck wrote about love between spouses, what it is and what it isn't, why we feel certain kinds of romantic love to be overwhelming and right. In discussing the basis for a sustained marriage, he painted an analogy that struck a chord. Peck likened marriage and a secure family life to the base camp for an even higher mountain climb. In mountaineering, a base camp represents the source of support, restoration, and supply—a shared effort dependent on all members of the group. Base camp provides a place to feel safe, secure, and protected.

By comparison, the mountain climb itself is based on individual effort, power, achievement, and a solidly personal effort—not a group endeavor. The two elements need to work hand in hand so all participants not only feel supported but also encourage each other's individual aspirations. That balance between group and personal needs can be hard to find, as it was in our marriage.

In too many marriages, Peck wrote, the husband climbs the mountain outside the home in the form of work or other achievements. He takes his base camp for granted and believes his money will provide the needed support. He expects base camp to serve him for his efforts devoted to his career while his wife runs it. This can breed resentment from a wife who feels neglected and not fully appreciated.

On the other hand, according to Peck, many wives think the base camp or family is their life's work and that their own aspirations must take second place. Subsequently, they not only exclude the husband from home life but bury whatever urges they may have for their own mountain climbing.

My wife and I didn't have this balance right at all. We both wanted to be bigger fixtures at "base camp" than was comfortable for the other person. My personal aspirations had turned as much inward as outward, a change that wasn't welcomed. And with barely being aware of it, we brought tons of emotional baggage from our own family histories into our conflict. Feeling justified and victimized by the other person, blaming each other became the easier road to take rather than examining our unconscious beliefs and changing the resulting dynamics.

Unfortunately, we fell into this sticky morass and failed in our efforts at resolving any of this dysfunction. We reluctantly agreed to separate. At this low, dark point, I felt devoid of any hope or light. As much as I acted like things would be better, especially with our five- and eight-year-old daughters, I felt as lost as I had ever been.

BEGINNING TO HEAL

The period immediately following our divorce, roughly ten years ago, was painful and confusing. Not only was I living alone again, but I couldn't interact with my daughters every day as I'd done for their entire lives. Although I had fought for more, I ended up seeing them slightly less than half the time. The separation was also painful for my daughters, who didn't understand the new arrangements. They simply trusted us when we said things would get better.

There was no getting around our family tragedy—one that has scarred each of us in some way. And each of us will continue to process the experiences in our psyches, our relations with others, and our present and future lives.

During that period, I found myself at the bottom of the rebuilding process that began on that train ride. The hell of hopelessness and self-blame I experienced following the divorce led to a long purgatorial climb into the light and an appreciation of life far beyond anything I'd expected. The two areas that my epiphany on the train made me prioritize—my daughters' well-being and my own health—became even more focused. Both became the anchors of my life, deeper than ever, and eventually led me out of that darkness.

The one upside was having extra time and space to be on my own, with and without my daughters. The absence of the daily angst and pressures I'd felt in the marriage allowed me to take a deep breath and more deeply understand this new world coming alive inside me. I could be as fully honest as my emotions and circumstances would let me.

During this period, I went back into psychotherapy to help me sort things out and be better aware of what my daughters were going through. I was also more spontaneous, candid, and involved with my daughters when they were with me—something our previous lifestyle had less room for. And I doubled down on my health research and practice, albeit with private sadness and solitude.

I'm not sure how I made it through the days when I wasn't with the girls. Still, I was learning firsthand the visceral, intertwined process of healing that addressed not only the physical but the mind and heart. I learned that the new scars trying to form couldn't, yet old scars had been ripped open and needed to be addressed. Those from my early life had mended badly, if at all. Healing had its work cut out for me.

The relentless, optimistic perseverance my daughters exhibited helped sustain me. They wanted to embrace life with all their youthful exuberance despite what had happened. They didn't ponder and worry like I did; they simply got on with seeking enjoyment in everything they did. In addition to my giving them the space and protection to be joyful, they took me along with them on their journey. Their playful exuberance provided a healing tonic for all of us, blessing us with lots of exploration, adventure, and fun.

Raising my daughters in these changed conditions and staying around as an active, healthy parent became more important than ever. That became my faith, the solid rock of action and meaning I returned to almost every day. I was also sustained by writing, by my deepening physical and increasing mind/body practice, and by a few trusted friends and teachers.

DESTINY, SUFFERING, AND RESILIENCE

At first, one of the worst emotions I felt was that I had failed as a father. My critical, fear-filled feelings colored my experience of life much of the time. This was intertwined with realizing that I blamed my own father for leaving me when he died.

Like my mother had been, I became a single parent with all the stigma and pain from that episode of my early life. The emotional intersection of the past and present became all too real in therapy sessions as well as in day-to-day life. I saw how the emotions in the timeless terrain of my subconscious affected my experiences in the present.

I feared for my children's future, thinking that somehow their fate would be similar to mine. Despite my intent to shield my daughters, they experienced suffering in their childhoods, and I was partly the agent of that suffering. Everything I'd wanted to avoid in my children's lives had happened on its own anyway; the secure family life I desired for them and myself—the one I never had—had fallen apart. How history repeats itself!

Yet I prayed they would not go through life as challenged as I was. I wanted them to feel more love along the way than I had, to have more support. How could I accomplish that?

THREE PATHS

The answers lay along three parallel paths: psychotherapy, my interconnected health practice, and the spiritual direction my inclinations and health studies steered me toward. I sensed being guided by a force I was learning to appreciate more. It had given me a kind of strength and resilience that helped navigate my way, albeit far from perfectly, until this point.

My therapist was also a child psychologist. Her help and insight provided the tools and advice to best love my daughters and give them what they need. This included self-love, something in short supply in my past.

Fostering my daughters' own ability to deal with adversity in the present and future became as important as my initial attempts at protecting them from it. When they were with me, they got my undivided attention—no phones or work. I signed up for as many school activities as I could to see them more often. I sought to let them express themselves, to become as fully genuine and wholehearted as possible. Their authentic feelings, even if uncomfortable and troubling, were welcomed, not feared. Most of all, I wanted them to know I loved them no matter what. *Their lives mattered*, not only to me but to themselves and the world at large. This sentiment differed distinctly from my own constricted upbringing.

WHAT BETTER GIFT

What better gift is there than to teach children how to be resilient in the face of life's challenges—to rely on their trusted inner guide, their unique inner voice, in the course of living and learning? As the song says, "God bless the child that's got his own."

Life dishes out many challenges—from teenage dramas to the kind of later life trials I'm navigating. Our trusted inner compass comes from an integrated inner life that, in turn, comes from being loved for who we are, not from how anyone wants us to be. Many religions place that guiding power *outside* us, yet I know it resides *inside*. I feel it flow through my veins. I can trust it to be a resource when I need it. Helping my children discover their own inner lives is all I want. The rest is window dressing.

No storms are their fault; feeling "not good enough" (as I did for much of my life) only makes things worse. No one ever became a good sailor in calm seas. Learning from life's storms makes us better able to deal with adversity and suffering. Yes, suffering is built in, as is resilience and recovery. But like exercise, by taxing ourselves, we become stronger. And through weathering storms, a big upside emerges.

9

The Great Guide

*"I used to feel like a boat,
completely at the mercy of
an ocean of thoughts that beat
against me one wave at a time.
Now I realize
I am not the boat
I am the ocean."*
—MELODY GOTTFRIED, *Self-Love Poetry*

"The one who bows and one who is bowed to are one."
—THICH NHAT HANH

What began as tentative first steps and a refocusing, accelerated and expanded after I experienced my own mortality. I aim to convey some of that experience in the chapters that follow. Yet this book wouldn't hold together without a further description of the other dimension that entered my awareness and became a big part of my journey.

Health is a gift I received at birth, a blessing for which no one—not my parents nor anyone else—was responsible. They may have been agents, but they didn't build the "hardware" that made it happen. Call it evolution, God, higher power, the infinite, providence, or any other name humans have given it in their attempt to define it since the dawn of consciousness, this power has evolved through a guiding universal spirit that not only created the universe and kept it evolving; it created the "rules" by which it runs. I sense this power as the wonder we feel inside when we contemplate our existence, think about life and death, and consult our conscience. Studying this power's depths and awe, history and future will keep humans going for a long, long time.

Religions past and present have claimed this kind of faith territory and probably do a better job acknowledging the mystery of existence than science does. But the myths and beliefs of religions only go so far. As Joseph Campbell extensively documented, coming to terms with our existence has been humans' work in thousands of versions for eons. Religions that are practiced today have their roots in books and stories thousands of years old and often require us to suspend new knowledge to conform to their beliefs and rituals.

In the period following my divorce, this ultimate power as I experienced it directly became a real presence. It has only grown inside me ever since, not only as a principal guiding force but as the subject of many interests, health related and otherwise. Acknowledging the guiding force's role was a big step for a lifelong nonbeliever like me. My belief doesn't fall within the lines of any one religion, but I can acknowledge the metaphors and strains of various religions along the way. I respect them as I've opened up to a vast and unexpected world within me—one that has enriched my life and understanding greatly.

TURNING TO PRAYER

When we get stuck, how do we fix ourselves? Ultimately, we want to take action. But before action comes inspiration from a source as mysterious as any other.

In the classic scene from *Zen and the Art of Motorcycle Maintenance*, Robert Pirsig describes how, by staring at a broken engine part for a long while and allowing his mind to go blank, his main character Phaedrus sees a solution "pop" into his mind. A broken emptiness gives way to an idea that will solve his problem.

Pirsig calls this act of going from broken to mended, of creating a solution from nothing, *quality*. And this same healing force inspires us to solve problems of our own. Many times we experience them as WTF moments or messages from God. They're certainly part of the wonder of the inner life I'm living today.

For example, many times I have gone to bed with either a specific problem or a feeling of being lost, and I've prayed for a solution. Who am I praying to? Any power that can help me—the forces of the universe. More often than not, a solution or direction pops into my head by the next morning. Sometimes it takes longer, yet my prayer is always heard. Is it heard *inside* me or *outside*? I don't know. But it dwells within me in the form of inspiration. *This vast power is the fundamental source of life and existence. And when I pray to it, I'm asking to be healed.*

I put my practicality and control aside, and I simply trust in the healing of this "universe" within me. Anne Lamott's wonderful book about prayer, *Help, Thanks, Wow: The Three Essential Prayers*, emphasizes that no matter what you believe in, some entity *out there* or *in here* can hear the word "help." Wheels turn, and it ultimately leads to solid ground when I trust it. For the more I let myself believe in an invisible, powerful, beneficial presence in life—a great guide—the more progress I make. When I feel negative toward myself, things don't work. When I feel positive, loved, cared for, and listened to—or even when I'm admittedly stuck and allow myself to feel that—everything works better.

The dynamics that shape how much I love myself exist *inside me* on a deeper subconscious level than I was used to seeing. They exist in the same place as dreams and biology, the parts that keep us healthy and alive. Very little about the process is rational or logical; it's almost entirely intuitive and visceral. This immensely beneficial work has been integral to how I experience life today.

THE UNIVERSAL QUEST

One of my best allies on this voyage into faith, spirit, and inner life has been Joseph Campbell, through his encyclopedic writings about the search for God throughout the history of our species. He has made the overwhelming case that, from our earliest days of conscious thought and when we could realize life was temporary and death will come, our ancestors wondered about existence. The history of religion reflects their attempts at defining and influencing these powers, of naming their gods and finding ways to get those gods to bless them.

In a book Campbell edited for his mentor Heinrich Zimmer, this four-word sentence reverberated deep inside me: "We can't borrow God."[1] That means the path to any spiritual understanding comes from inside, from soul searching, or from despair, curiosity, anxiety, or any number of genuine human emotions. God, or what he calls the "divine Transcendent Principle," must be found anew by each person journeying through life. It's just like children who need to arrive at their own version of personhood if they are to be genuinely themselves and not copies of others. This principle can never be conveyed by another; it only comes from direct internal experience. That means religion and faith can't be copied and still claim to be the real thing.

This includes the teachings of all the world's religions—all of them products of the individual religion founders' personal discovery of God. And this goes for every religion currently practiced on the planet as well as every so-called pagan religion. They are the products of our ancestors trying to understand the universe and help themselves in doing so.

Many great lessons are conveyed in these religions, including from Judaism in my own early life. Yet they all need to be put through the fire of personal experience and belief in order to become inner guideposts instead of rote practices dictated by words on a page. To the extent I follow the rules and practices of religions of old, as beneficial as they can be, I could miss out on the fundamental process of coming to terms with my infinite self—in my own life and times. That's the difference between *knowing* God in my head and *experiencing* God in my bones.

GRACE AND SERENDIPITY

In *The Road Less Traveled*, Peck wrote about grace and serendipity as forces that aren't entertained enough in modern life—especially in modern psychology. While I remain a believer in many of the benefits of science and rational thought, my study brings me face-to-face with the limits of purely academic and "provable" knowledge.

Exploring life through what goes on in the 90 percent of my mind and body that's nonrational and below the surface has given me a great deal of peace and understanding. Very little is rational and logical in that sphere. Rather, it's a world of poetry and dreams and music as well as flesh and blood and guts, all of which bring me the gift of life every day.

Mostly, *how I feel inside* determines the life I lead. This steady, wonderful feeling was something I rarely experienced until now. My other life that was concerned with external achievement and admiration—how I am perceived by others—is still part of me. But it's only *part* of me, not my reason to exist. Each of us has a personal self as well as a universal self. The universal self is the 90 percent of us that runs the show, the operating system under the surface. Acknowledging its power has caused a shift inside of me that has changed everything.

The quality of my new life defies description because it's mostly radiantly visceral, not cerebral. Call it joy, serenity, wonder, depth, grace, clarity, coherence, harmony, contentment, purpose, synergy, bliss, or any number of words—it's an oceanic feeling of belonging and being part of this amazing universe. It's also feeling entitled to live genuinely, wholeheartedly—the experience of being the *essence of love* for myself and others.

PART II

My Life Practice

A New Definition of Health

"I Sing the Body Electric."

—WALT WHITMAN

"The miracle of life is life itself."

—ANONYMOUS

Given all I have learned and with increasing confidence as I refined my own practice, I began to formulate a comprehensive definition of health for myself. It has come out of my experimentation and is backed up by trusted metrics that include everything from modern medical tests to visceral emotions and judgment. So far, I have been blessed with a high degree of later-life health and vitality. I'm learning to navigate conflicting and self-serving advice by enhancing my own inner compass, which has become a 24/7 preoccupation that I thrive on.

My health starts with the firm belief that it is *my* responsibility, only outsourced to others as I choose. Just like saying, "You can't borrow God," you can't borrow health by doing what someone else recommends. This includes a subtle mix of what I want, what makes sense, what feels right, and what can be measured. I treat my body and brain as an integrated organism with all parts connected to and affecting every other part. It's how nature made me.

When my biological, mental, and spiritual health don't balance well with each other, I usually feel unease, anxiety, or physical discomfort. Where does the boundary exist between a thought or feeling and a biochemical reaction in my brain or body? No one knows, at least not yet. The ample evidence of how belief affects physical health shows the mystery to be a persistent fly in the ointment of current medical theory. The more I work at it, though, the softer the boundaries become between these often mislabeled "separate" realms. I try to keep my inner life and my biological life in sync with each other. Fixing one usually helps the other.

What helps me feel alive and healthy every day? What sustains me, keeps me energetic and curious, enables me to be productive and positively involved with myself and others? The intricate, miraculous visceral combination of chemistry and biology within me. My heart beats, my blood flows, my brain thinks, and all my senses kick in. The entire system works together because of the miracle of life.

When I perceive something external that is beautiful or fun or sad or funny, my sensory body enables me to appreciate it. Tending to this flame is the foundation and my top priority. Ninety percent or more of the energy I expend goes to the vast underground within me and the source of my health. For instance, I spend most mornings appreciating the force that sustains me. First, I lie in bed and value waking up. I breathe deeply. I empty my mind as much as I can to keep it visceral, not mental. I want to *feel* the life inside me.

Then I take a heart rate variability (HRV) reading and do breathing exercises such as the Wim Hof Method or the "low and slow" methods advocated by Patrick McKeown in *The Oxygen Advantage*. I focus on my body, the amazing complexity and wonder of how I've slept and been restored. I follow this with a morning cup of tea and fifteen to thirty minutes of movement, stretching, and gentle yoga.

All the while, I'm continuing to appreciate the universe for the gift of movement, the gift of breath. I feel the oxygen deep in my bones, joints, muscles, organs, and lungs while sensing the benefits of circulation being transferred to all parts of my body.

This routine contrasts to how I spent mornings in my previous life. They were filled with plans, worries, and expectations, usually rushed and frenetic. Being acutely sensitive to timing and schedules, I worried about being on time. Waking up the way I do now resets me and whatever lies ahead that day. Not only have I eliminated or lessened what used to be troubling—letting them go as nonessentials—but those that remain become more manageable with self-appreciation and gratitude. A favorite Wayne Dyer quotation is this: "If you change the way you look at things, the things you look at will change."

THE GOLDEN AGE OF HUMAN EVOLUTION

As noted earlier, a foundation of my new definition of health is our evolutionary history. How the universe made us into what we are plays a huge part in how I practice health.

Our modern time on earth represents less than one thousandth of a percent of total human time. Before that, our ancestors were hunter-gatherers. Fresh natural food, constant movement, and rhythms guiding the natural universe were integral to their existence and survival. *That* is the life our bodies were made for. *That* is the golden age of human evolution.

For most of that time, how humans interacted with the world and stayed healthy remained the same. We were part of the landscape, guided by our instincts to survive in synchronicity with our surroundings. Our bodies and immune systems evolved accordingly but still operate on the same rhythms and principles developed back then. The past fifty thousand years of our consciousness, language, art, technology, and knowledge has been a blip in evolutionary time.

This golden age of evolution wasn't only physical. Our ancestors were evolving instincts, emotions, and new behaviors to complement their changing bodies. The challenges and threats they confronted provided the groundwork for evolving new capabilities, both physical and mental. Nature made us a seamless tapestry of feeling, thought, biochemistry, and electricity as well as flesh, blood, and bone. Instincts still guide much of our daily lives. Any separation is pure illusion, for our bodies operate as an organic whole, not separate parts thrown together.

Today, I believe we're living a maladapted version of that life (or "mismatched" in the words of Daniel Lieberman). Like Cinderella's stepsisters trying to stuff their large feet into an elegant glass slipper, we experience our bodies as modern versions of *what we think they ought to be*, not the rugged evolutionary survival machines they *are*.

For example, we tend to think of healing as a process that only kicks in when we get sick or injured; it's our body's reaction to something being out of balance. And while the human body does go into a higher gear during injury or disease, it's in a constant state of maintenance—ceaselessly repairing, cleaning, digesting, growing, repelling invaders, making energy, regulating, balancing, and renewing. When our daily healing level dips in strength, our immune system weakens, but it still works 24/7. It's more than an ambulance rescuing us when we get sick!

ACTIVE HEALING AND LIFE FORCE

Active healing is synonymous with life force: *the deep mystery of the healthy functioning of everything within*. Aligning with this force is the goal of my health practice.

Each of us has a homeostatic equilibrium that's more than a simple biological formula. It ties to our core conception of who we are, how loved we are, how we can survive, and our life experiences to this point. It can be a setting that resists change *because* we've been this way for so long and survived, although not perfectly. We feel safe and protected, even if we aren't as conscious about our health as we could be. Moving this homeostatic needle is the real mark of living a healthier life.

My journey has taught me that good health is something I hadn't fully experienced before, but it also differs from comfort. Again, I define good health as being vibrant, energetic, alive, and in harmony with my aspirations. It's the level of health I was exposed to after my first detox. No longer is it the province of endless advice and measurements such as how far or fast I can walk, how much weight I can lift, what my cholesterol readings and blood tests show, and what my body mass index measures. In conversations with others, particularly older people, I'm not sure they realize how it feels to be in good health as I define it. To the extent they outsource their health to doctors and others, they're defining their degree of health by what's on their medical chart.

For me, good health also means accepting and appreciating its power inside me and enjoying its benefits. It's about taking responsibility and caring for myself, loving myself, feeling grateful for healing and health—the sum of everything that sustains me. Health is the naturally occurring state the universe means for me to experience.

And when I'm not feeling healthy, I feel that too. Ill health can range from low energy to discomfort or increased inflammation and anxiety. It could be realizing something new inside, often preceded by increased stress. Symptoms can have physical as well as emotional sources; they can be addressed with both physical resources (such as therapeutic yoga) and emotional resources (such as psychotherapy, prayer, meditation, intention, and more).

THE CULPRIT KNOWN AS INFLAMMATION

In my studies, inflammation has appeared as the culprit behind many diseases and conditions that curtail the quality and length of our lives. It has been linked to heart conditions, diabetes, arthritis, cancer, poor digestion, autoimmune disease, and other problems of aging. And like many words about health being popularized through Dr. Google, "inflammation" is much misunderstood.

Inflammation is a highly complex biochemical process that ranges from restricted blood flow to swelling to increased mucous and other bodily effects. It's also the body reacting to a form of stress or toxin or invader. As the first phase of healing, inflammation kicks the immune system into high gear to stabilize and repair what's causing the problem.

Having short-term inflammation is normal, and it goes away naturally once the body repairs itself. As an example, after I've exercised, lactic acid builds up in my muscles before they start to heal, and they rebuild slightly stronger than they were before. I sense it as stiffness. When I did my first detox, I felt inflammation in my joints and sinuses. Today, I feel it when I get sick and also when I am anxious. It could also be due to indigestion or a headache. Many studies back up the link between physical symptoms and stress, tension, or anxiety. Inflammation has emotional as well as physical triggers. Whatever its source, it makes me feel out of sorts.

Modern lifestyles deliver a cornucopia of inflammation triggers as well as diversions that keep us from realizing them as such. Whether it be from toxic processed foods and lack of movement, or schedules, expectations, and fears that come with all sorts of internal and external pressures, low-level inflammation has become omnipresent and often disguised. But rather than follow the advice it's giving us—to pay better attention and take action—we tend to treat the symptom rather than the underlying cause so we can "get on with our lives." This happens with anything from pain relievers to caffeine to alcohol to illusions about what is actually wrong. Yet inflammation's underlying cause rarely goes away.

Take digestion problems such as Crohn's disease or irritable bowel disease (IBD). The underlying condition for these is usually an imbalance in the gut affecting the lining of the colon or small intestine. The cause could be a weak or imbalanced microbiome, a steady diet of toxic or sugary foods, and/or a subconscious emotional link.

In today's medical world, a traditional doctor would prescribe anti-inflammatory or "beta-blocker" drugs so the symptoms don't flare up. The drugs themselves, though, might affect the immune system's natural balance in keeping itself healthy. By comparison, a functional or integrative medical doctor would look deeper into the cause of the condition. (Would either one examine the role of underlying emotions in treating the problem?)

I have suffered regular (but temporary) mild indigestion and irritable bowel syndrome. Relief came when I linked them to my state of mind or some increased anxiety. I also rebalanced my digestive system with anti-inflammatory foods and probiotics. In many cases, I felt immediate relief when I made the connection to an inner emotional truth.

The goal of health should be to *return to a natural drug-free state* and not depend on drugs for "reduced-symptom" living. I'm not making a case against acute medical care with antibiotics and other drugs for short-term fixes. But overtinkering with our immune system by regularly using drugs has the long-term effect of weakening the body's ability to diagnose and repair itself. It's like believing a pesticide we use will only kill the insects we don't like.

THE ROLE OF RESILIENCE

In all my studies and practice, I keep coming back to something I read in *The Longevity Project* by Howard Friedman and Leslie Martin. At eight decades, it has the longest span of any longevity study out there. What's more, it focuses on all aspects of one's lifestyle, including psychology. Spoiler alert: a few paragraphs near the end of the book sum up a key finding of this study. It states:

> Across the life span, many predictors emerged as to who would do better and who would do worse, who would live longer and who would die younger. It was not good cheer or being popular and outgoing that made the difference. It was not those who took life easy, played it safe, or avoided stress who lived the longest. Rather, it was those who—through an often-complex pattern of persistence, prudence, hard work, and close involvement with friends and communities—headed down meaningful, interesting life paths and, as we have illustrated, found their way back to these healthy paths each time they were pushed off the road.[1]

As important as diet and movement is to dealing with life's detours, so is using resilience to overcome challenges. Nature has made me stronger and kept me evolving via resilience. And when I promote my own health to stay strong and vital for as long as possible, I'm challenging myself and my body to provoke nature's healing power. This, too, is health. Someone once said, "Life is a marathon; you've got to train for it." Thus, health and longevity in later life is an *ultramarathon* and requires even more training. For me, that means inducing, encouraging, and appreciating the healing powers nature provided me.

MODERN MEDICINE AND SELF-CARE

Modern Western medicine has brought much with it such as acute care and interventionist measures to combat disease and dysfunction. Yet by outsourcing our health to modern medicine, we have discarded much of the wisdom and practice of prevention—the sound, nature-driven practices that have kept humans alive and steadily advancing for millions of years.

The worst aspects of our modern health care system involve a closed loop. We get sick on processed food diets, lack of movement, and boredom with life, and then go to a doctor to get artificially "cured" or maintained on prescription drugs. Many people live in a state of ignorance about their own biology, their true inner power, and their dependence on consumer medical culture. I witness this especially in older people who tend to accept the definitions of others rather than feeling their own power to embrace their later years in all their wonder.

Even though modern medicine would like to take credit for curing us, nature ultimately does. Modern medicine can remove or reduce the obstacles to the body's natural ability to heal in many ways. For example, its adherents administer antibiotics, surgically remove cancer cells, and scrape plaque from an artery. Yet, what provides the *ultimate* healing once those procedures are done? Nature. We largely take for granted that well-practiced medicine *assists* the natural process but doesn't *replace* it. Even a vaccine, a wonder of preventive medical science, relies on the body's natural immunity to fight off a small dose of disease and develop resistance to it.

For the most part, functional or integrative medicine does a better job at prevention than interventionist medicine. At least natural foods and movement are part of their prescriptions for health. Traditional medicine, though, is slowly catching on. As Dr. Mark Hyman said, "Someday all of medicine will be under the same umbrella, prevention as well as treatment."

Yet even functional medicine isn't as comprehensive and integrated as I would like because it relies on the same dependent doctor-patient relationship. We need more self-care to truly have a healthier population. For example, in selecting my healthcare providers, I keep our relationships as collaborative as possible and don't blindly follow their advice. Rather, I weigh their recommendations as information to consider while relying on my own research, instincts, and goals.

HEALTH AND CARE

It seems "health" and "care" have always been synonymous. Nature has programmed us to care for others, especially our children, when they are sick or injured. So strong is the association of feeling better with parental care that, in my own childhood, I believed my mother held the power to heal me when I was sick. Blind faith in that power contributes to the hold on outsourcing our health to doctors so strong. The common thread is this: *Care both from others and ourselves is a vital part of healing.* This applies to prevention as well as curing.

Conversely, when we cut ourselves and the wound gets inflamed, for example, why do we say that it looks "angry"? Perhaps the inflammation at the root of so many diseases I want to avoid has a relationship with anger and disapproval?

In her book *CURE*, Jo Marchant points to studies that show the amount of time doctors spend with their patients has a dramatic effect on how they respond to treatment. This makes complete sense considering how I felt as a child—that is, believing someone else holds that power. In truth, however, only *nature* holds that power. Yet, how much I care about myself and/or am cared for by others enhances the process.

In fact, realizing I was in charge of my own health set me on this journey. I began taking more responsibility for my health as opposed to seeking outside care. For me, health has become synonymous with self-love. Part of my journey also deals with uncovering the hidden sources of self-hate within me, dynamics that are long suppressed features of my childhood.

Indeed, advice on health provided by others doesn't produce the same passion to take action as my inner callings do. Largely self-sustaining, these callings get reinforced through positive feedback and results. Practicing health as I do is not a quick fix. Rather, it relies on a different rhythm and more subtle awareness than taking pills or visiting doctors. This approach has generated many benefits along the way, as discussed in detail in Part III.

MY RADICAL LONGEVITY MISSION

My new definition of health calls for encouraging nature's miraculous healing power to keep repairing and renewing within me. That means doing naturally what radical research programs in juventology (the study of youth) are doing to find answers using drugs and other therapies. Scientists such as Aubrey de Grey and his SENS Research Foundation have identified many of the same life-giving pathways to learn how our bodies restore themselves. They want to enhance these healing pathways with medical intervention to slow aging. While viable solutions are years away, I'm pursuing my own version of enhancing this eons-old health system with natural methods.

As I get older, being in charge of my health requires even more effort than when I was younger. And because I'm interested in radical longevity, my dedication to researching methods needs to be radical as well. The systems that have supported me weaken as I get older. Then I think how any hardship I endure is miniscule compared to what our ancestors lived through. The payoff in maintaining my health has been and will be worth every second of extra effort.

MY PLAN FOR HEALTH AND LIFE

Again, my goal is to keep functioning powerfully for as long as possible. It's not about staying as strong as I once was (although I have so far). Ultimately, it's about staying as strong and healthy as I'm *capable* of. That calls for experimenting with different methods, techniques, and practices. Yes, one day my health will decline and my time will come. But until then, I intend to thrive.

My plan is like a mission statement that evolves and changes. A full health cornerstone gives shape to my daily activities and prioritizes them. These priorities are:

1. My children's welfare
2. My welfare as it pertains to my children and the quality of my experiences
3. The continued expression, realization, and freedom of my curiosity and spirit. That requires health, inspiration, and time. Any notions of status, wealth, and image have fallen into the background.

Derived from these priorities are my goals from the categories of practice and training:

1. Power
2. Fuel or nutrition
3. Movement, motion, and flexibility
4. Balance, alignment, and posture
5. Recovery, renewal, and inspiration
6. Clarity
7. Metrics, diagnosis, healing, and support

(Part II explores each of these categories individually.)

Each category interacts, balances, harmonizes with, and supports all the others. Together, they form a whole like a steel cable made of many strands. For example, balance is a product of strength, flexibility, and awareness, and it provides a good gauge of how these aspects are working together.

None of these categories is more important than any other with one possible exception—power—because it supports and flows through all the others. Different combinations come to my attention as I practice. Like an orchestra and all its instruments, the components depend on a complex harmony of inner and outer circumstances. My body is no less complicated than a magnificent symphony—and no less beautiful to experience.

Specific exercises and diet support each category. Just as important is the awareness that comes from having love and emotional support. To the extent a physical problem needs attention or a future ailment needs prevention, my focus derives from awareness, inner strength, compassion, conviction, purpose, physical practice, and change in lifestyle. Emotional resistance and historic patterns play their parts as well.

At the core is a presence made up of conscience, soul, gut, center, providence, the universe, or God—all providing a deep inner connection. This presence is something I rely on to guide me. When life is flowing, I have the clarity I'm seeking. At other times, I'm challenged to experience life as I want to. When that happens, finding my way through the challenge is as essential to my health as any other part of life.

THE ROLE OF BELIEF

Many current evidence-based studies, even those advocating only diet and exercise, exclude how we feel about ourselves—perhaps the most important part of being healthy. Any discussion or study that fails to take personal factors into account misses the point. In my work, I use the terms "emotional biology" or "psychophysical" to describe this integration. As stated, health is a condition of *overall* well-being, not just physical well-being. It enables us to enjoy a *genuine* life, one we want to be living. How we feel about our lives and our state of health are integral to each other. As Joseph Campbell writes, "The privilege of a lifetime is being who you are." *If we're not feeling that way, something is off.*

Don't get me wrong. I'm not dismissing the value of knowing my blood pressure or cholesterol or nutrient levels or any other diagnostic tool. Yet while I've included medical information in my definition of health, no medical chart has a box for "clarity" or "resilience" or "balance."

"How is your life?" is a question doctors ought to ask in any diagnosis. Until they do, we need to ask it of ourselves. The Japanese word *ikigai* has many meanings, but ultimately it conveys a reason to get up every morning.

I'm especially struck by health and longevity studies that don't factor in a belief element. Books like *The Blue Zones* focus on mimicking the lifestyles of people in places where longevity goals are achieved. But what those people eat and how they live must also include the fact that they've seen their relatives live to a great age. As a result, these people *expect* to live that long too. They feel contentment and love and respect for themselves. These beliefs are in their bones. I'm convinced these kinds of feelings and beliefs play an outsized role that's overlooked in many of our current health practices.

At age seventy-three, I am smack in the heart of my later years, although I feel and move better in many ways than I did twenty years ago. I'd like to keep going strong for another thirty years. How I feel about my time to come has every bearing on how I live those years. And achieving that goal will be affected by my beliefs, my state of mind, and my ability to practice being healthy. If I see my remaining years as being full of decline and frailty, I'm doomed. If I see them as vibrant and anticipate full enjoyment, my entire outlook shifts. *This core belief is as vital to my health as any other factor.*

The practices I include in Part II have worked for me after much trial and error, and they may resonate for you. They're based on my journey toward health as *I* define it.

No matter your age and lifestyle, health is a vital factor in your quality of life as you get older, so don't accept others' definitions or you'll be robbed of being genuine, wholehearted, and living without regret.

Consider my ideas for navigating your health issues in the chapters that follow, and choose those that fit for *you* as you manage your own lifelong health journey.

10

Power and Its Cousins
Energy, Strength, Endurance, and Vitality

"The human body is sustained by the same prana that nourishes the universe."

—JOHN HOLLAND

What I call "power" has a special place in the qualities of well-being, for only one eternal source of power or energy exists in this universe and flows through all of us. This force enables us to heal, grow, learn, transcend, transform, change, move, and get stronger. It is the source of wonder and curiosity as well as what made our bodies what they are.

The same power that created a trillion suns also created human beings over evolutionary eons. We are born with power in abundance, packed into our single-cell embryo self. The blueprint of who we are (provided we get enough care in early life) contains everything we'll need to be alive. It's the ultimate answer that mystical and mythic heroes sought on their quests—from Buddha to Jesus to those who are still seeking.

I feel power within me as energy, strength, endurance, love, passion, and curiosity. When it's present in my here and now, my system works better. When it's absent or obscured, my quality of life deteriorates. As I have learned, this power thrives in me when I love and accept myself and don't blame or judge myself. Yet even when it's not immediately accessible, I know it's quietly humming in the 90 percent of me that keeps me healthy. I see it in our immense galaxy with all its stars and planets, and I see it in the smallest microbe. Even subatomic particles flash their quantum energy on and off according to the rhythm of their power.

We tend to think of this force as primarily manifesting in our bodies as strength and physical endurance. Yet it also makes up the qualities we call grit, determination, resilience, fortitude, illumination, love, patience, anger, hate, avarice, jealousy, and competition. All these inner aspects interact with and are part of my physical being in many ways, both obvious and subtle. For example, professional athletes say that once they've mastered the physical part of their sport, their actual performance lies in their inner world and emotions. And that makes the difference!

Harnessing the synergy of this power enables athletes to transcend their physical skill, endurance, and strength. It's called "being in the zone," and together with belief, this synergy is more important than any other aspect of their sport. I suspect this is the underlying reason watching sports remains popular. We witness the sheer wonder of seeing this extraordinary human capability at the peak of its powers. (I also believe we would have a healthier society if more fans moved and sought this power as much as athletes do.) And not accidentally, most professional sports revolve around movements that were important in prehistoric years, including throwing, hitting, running, and teamwork.

ABILITY TO MOVE FORWARD

Power also refers to our ability to move forward, to overcome, to be resilient, to transcend circumstances, to do better today than yesterday. We strive for it on some level, yet it also visits without even trying. Its work can never be fully completed or understood.

Power is the flip side of entropy or laziness. Even though entropy exists in my universe at times, I have found it to be part of recovering and healing, the parasympathetic phase of what goes on inside me. It allows me to have "nothing to do." I used to criticize myself for this apparent laziness. Now I accept it as an essential part of recovery, healing, and inspiration. Effort always returns, usually eclipsing previous levels. I believe this transcending force is part of the underlying rhythm of every part of the universe woven into the fabric of space and time—and especially the fabric of *us*. Physicists can explain what makes this power tick, whether it's black holes, dark energy, or dark matter. I am content to simply *feel* it.

Ultimately, my practice is devoted to maintaining and increasing this power in all its forms. Call it motivation, gumption, guts, life force, knowledge, patience, wisdom, strength, or any other name—*power impels me toward health as the force that keeps me alive.*

Simply acknowledging and respecting power and then allowing it into my world has changed me immeasurably. Blocking power, not experiencing it clearly, or trying to control or deny it remains in my past. Thinking I don't deserve to be blessed by this force at one time was tragic. Letting go of that criticism and trusting it to guide me has significantly improved my life. How? It has resulted in increased physical strength as well as enhanced mental and spiritual energy. Hopefully, it has also freed up blockages that might have led to disease down the road.

AS PEOPLE AGE

As we age, we tend to believe that our vitality quantitatively lessens over time. We accept false information as established belief. More than that, we assume we *will* get weaker and believe it when people say, "That's just aging." Yet these beliefs accelerate physical decline!

Much of the current experience of aging and health is based on beliefs that studies have shown to be wrong. A good example is neuroscientist Daniel Levitin's book *Successful Aging* in which he scientifically debunks commonly held notions about losing capacity as we age. Not true. Exercise, diet, and other lifestyle factors make up part of the battle to challenge these erroneous beliefs. Equally important is exploring my inner life by defining what I want and facing what stands in the way.

A LESSON ABOUT POWER

Years ago while planning a business trip to New York, I learned that Nikki Costello, my longtime yoga teacher, would be offering a one-day yoga retreat the day after I arrived. I signed up with trepidation knowing I'd feel jet lagged and probably wouldn't make it through the day. For whatever reason, though, I knew it was important to attend and be in supportive company. Little did I know I would receive a great gift.

After a full day of travel from London, I managed to get six hours of sleep before waking up at two a.m. New York time (my usual seven a.m. London time). The retreat would start in seven hours, so I wrote and read to pass the time. My stomach was empty, but I wasn't hungry, so when I arrived at the session, I was already tired and depleted. I told Nikki that if I crashed and left early, I was sorry and explained why. She smiled and replied, "Do what you can. I appreciate that you are here."

Nikki started by outlining the purpose of the retreat: *to find rest within the yoga practice and the balance point between exertion and relaxation, especially in our breathing.* We discussed that same purpose as it applies to finding peace and repose in our daily lives. When she said we would work hard in the morning's retreat and taper off in the afternoon, I groaned inside. *Just what I need in my state!* I thought. *But whatever happens, happens. Just go with it.*

The three-hour morning segment, based on Iyengar yoga, was harder than any yoga session I'd had. We did several poses and held them for what seemed like forever. In each pose, Nikki reinforced how to find the *nonstrenuous* aspect of that posture called the repose. She gave us these instructions:

- Ask, "Where in the pose are you not putting effort?"
- Ask, "Are you tightening muscles that aren't necessary to support yourself?"
- Only use the parts of your body you need to do the pose, and relax the other parts. Don't overuse those that are doing the work.
- Relax your jaw and tongue. Don't clench your teeth. They aren't necessary to support you.
- Make sure everything is aligned, and your body will support itself.
- Find the balance within the pose.

OPEN THE DOORWAY TO POWER

About an hour into the morning, something came alive in me that I'd never experienced before—a serene energy that kept me going the rest of the day. Not only could I hold the poses I already knew for a long time; I did other poses such as elbow stand that I hadn't been able to do before. I felt a sense of balance between exertion and rest, both being equally active, as if a doorway had opened into a new world like Dorothy opening the door to Oz.

This retreat experience changed my belief about yoga and energy. Despite doing a practice for more than twenty years, *what yoga means* and *where it could lead me* shifted forever that day. It isn't just an expenditure of energy physically; it's a complete experience of my "inner" life in the moment, a microcosm of universal energy. I now strive for this kind of energy balance in my life and my practice every day.

INNER SOURCE OF POWER

What is the source of my power? Where did that energy I experienced in class come from? Not from rest, willpower, or belief, nor from ideas I had previously used to explain internal energy. For sure, it didn't spring from caffeine, sugar, fat, protein, or any food or drug. My power seemed to come out of nowhere!

As a result, I had to suspend my belief that energy is directly associated with diet, sleep, or anything else. They all play their parts but are *not* the driving center. It was a "humble" energy I couldn't take credit for because I knew it had visited me. It wasn't power *over* anything or even mere willpower. Rather, it was serendipitous—an unexpected example of grace. I showed up at class to engage while leaving behind the judging part of me. *I simply stopped trying.*

My experience that day showed me an inner force that transcended my current state of understanding. Because of its strength and clarity, I knew I could arrive at a deeper, clearer place and understand this vital aspect of power in a new way.

My question then became "what can I do in my daily practice

to open these channels and get more of this kind of energy in my life?" Exploring answers to this question provides the backdrop of the chapters that follow. Whether from movement, exercise, writing, meditation, diet, contemplation, or psychotherapy, I'm cultivating energy that's at the heart of my quest to live longer and stay healthy. When I gain clarity in the presence of this life force and feel it *in my bones*, tasks become easier and I face obstacles with more facility. I am intensely alive and at ease with myself, and I feel more engaged, patient, and attentive with others. I'm sure this energy also affects my physical health.

TRANSFORMING EXISTING LIMITS

The evolution I've become so fascinated with is about transcending limits. Internally, this force shows up as *clarity*—the seemingly otherworldly visit of an idea or solution that didn't exist before, as my train ride and the yoga session exemplify. *All inner growth is the product of this power, a universal force available to anyone.*

Under its influence, answers and inspiration can appear as if by magic, given the time and space to do its work. It's what Robert Pirsig was getting at in *Zen and the Art of Motorcycle Maintenance*. He saw the solution to fixing his broken engine as a manifestation of this driving universal force. *Quality* had visited him and made its presence known.

Yes, power never rests; it drives everything.

Effort and Recovery

I have experienced two distinct and equally important phases with power—dynamic and static. Just as a muscle needs to heal and strengthen beyond its previous capability, we need to digest and appreciate the experience of power for it to feel at home within us. This mirrors the sympathetic and parasympathetic aspects of our autonomic nervous system. It's the same duality formed in every breath and heartbeat: *effort and recovery, effort and recovery.*

Power increases most when it's challenged, stressed, or made to overcome resistance, like a tree that grows taller when forced to seek the sunlight. That power helps ensure the tree's chances of survival. Similarly, movement provides a good example of this power at work. In ancestral times, hunger drove us to find food, making us move a great deal just to eat. Every day required meeting challenges like climbing a tree, pulling a root, or hunting an animal.

Hunting and gathering have provided the blueprint for what we can do for ourselves today. Walking, climbing, digging, pulling, throwing, and lifting—guided by our minds and senses and fueled by need—make up what our ancestors did for millions of years. Today, we don't challenge ourselves nearly enough, rarely exercising our resilience and strength. In our society, we have become weak, soft, and out of balance. This imbalance is the source of many modern physical ailments as well as alienations and misbeliefs.

POWER FREES UP RESOURCES

Cultivating integrated power is often missing in health and longevity advice. But when properly exerted and challenged, power begets more power. It frees up previously hidden resources and channels of energy.

I call my search for this power a work in progress—one that regularly transforms to accommodate new inputs and energy shifts. My body, mind, and spirit all need this attention to thrive. Combining the physical *and* existential elements of power has enhanced my health in deeper ways than dealing with them separately. I live as a whole organism, not separate parts. Having strong muscles and eating a good diet aren't enough to guarantee health or quality of life. The life force within me ultimately provides lasting health and meaning. The qualities of spirit, balance, harmony, and coordination come together to give me energy for the next inevitable challenge.

Most of all, *my connection with power allows me to be my truest self, living as wholeheartedly as I can.* This, in turn, spurs me to want to live a long time, stay healthy, and passionately enjoy being alive.

11

Fuel
What Keeps Us Operating

"You are what your body DOES with what you eat."
—GARY TAUBES

For virtually all our existence as human beings, getting enough nourishment to stay alive has been a constant challenge. Raw hunger, our most basic preprogrammed DNA-driven instinct, drives everything else. Our bodies need fuel to operate. Along with survival and reproduction, hunger drives the entire universe of living organisms. In the past, we had to move to eat. We learned what was good by using our senses—how things tasted and smelled, and how they made us feel. We ate anything edible, including bugs and worms and all sorts of leaves, plants, and other animals.

As we evolved, our bodies developed defenses including strong immune systems and hydrochloric acid in our stomachs to help deal with pathogens. We began to use tools and other skills in our quest to find food. What we settled on tasted good (or at least not bad) and was always natural, including the trillions of healthy bacteria that came along with it. The amount we had to move to gather or hunt this food and get at the edible parts (nut cracking, dead animal skinning, and hard chewing) ensured our bodies stayed efficient.

It was the perfect system—hunger and movement—to provide the fuel necessary for evolution and reproduction. Nature's perfect evolutionary DNA laboratory has made us who we are.

NUTRITION STARTING POINT

My starting point for nutrition goes back to the 99.99 percent of how we existed before agriculture and modern living. This history caused my body to consume what I needed, what was "good" for me, which included nutritional hunger, almost constant and varied movement, and a challenge to survive every day.

Today, I find my body works better when I eat less (and as directly from nature as possible) and when I move more. As a result of re-experiencing this primal energy, I have more energy, am thinner and lighter, and my belly feels emptier compared to before I lived like this. I also have less inflammation, more digestive comfort, and increased immune function.

Convincing research (see studies on diet cited in Resources) about diet and health includes a dramatic improvement in all blood markers, energy levels, and metabolic functions when people with disease-prone indicators are eating modern diets but switch to simple, fresh, mainly plant-based foods. Within a few weeks, they have lost weight and decreased their blood sugar, cholesterol, and inflammation. They feel better! I had the same effects when I did my detox. Now I say, "If it doesn't look like food, or if it comes in a box, package, container, or bottle, or if it was refined or processed from its natural state or made in a factory, I stay away from it."

Every study I read, or program or documentary I watch (see list in Resources) points to the same close-to-universal truth. Yet few of them credit the role of healing in the process. What are the effects on our bodies when we stop stuffing them with irritants and toxins found in modern diets? From my detox I learned that changing my diet allowed my body to start healing *and* to better digest my food. It could more fully absorb the many beneficial nutrients I was eating. In the process, the natural sensitivity and balance of my immune system was restored.

WHEN HEALTHY PEOPLE EAT A MODERN DIET

These same studies are true in reverse; when healthy people who follow traditional nonmodern diets shift to a modern processed food diet, they are less healthy. They could come from a Blue Zone like Okinawa where people live actively into their nineties and more. Or they could have a hunter-gatherer lifestyle like the Hadza in Tanzania or the Aboriginals in Australia. Yet, within a short period of eating a modern diet, all their health markers—blood pressure, glucose levels, cholesterol, weight, energy levels—worsen. They move less as well. With this shift, they markedly increase their chances of heart disease, diabetes, metabolic syndrome, and other diseases. They also increase their risks of dying earlier than when their diets were "clean." (For an extreme example, watch Morgan Spurlock's documentary *Super Size Me*, which describes what happened when he spent a month eating nothing but McDonald's food.)

The natural diets of people in these studies were culturally different, yet they all had one thing in common: no processed foods, fast foods, prepared foods, sugar, caffeine, alcohol, and manufactured fats or oils. They also had no rules on when or how to eat. They allowed their bodies, not their social habits, to dictate mealtimes and snack times—even skipping meals.

The relationship between food and blood test markers is as plain to see as any other truth about health. A healthy diet and its tag-team partner, movement, are the drivers of improved lipid, glucose, blood pressure, inflammation, and other markers. These are the essential elements in weight loss and weight increase, as well as the starting point for a range of metabolic diseases from arthritis to diabetes.

In my view of our modern diet, the choices of what and when to eat are self-serving and often just plain wrong. In our choices, we feel pressured by advertising, misinformation, social conventions, and even habits and tastes from our childhoods. We are the unaware, unquestioning, and unhealthy victims of this pressure, much of which comes from inside us.

METABOLIC BALANCE AND HEALING

In these studies, the predominant "quick change" in their subjects' lives is diet. But as valid as that looks, the people being studied underwent other changes that went unnoticed by the researchers. That is, when people improve their diets and start to feel better, a shift happens inside. As healing and a better metabolic balance come into play, they start caring for themselves and their health more than before. Not only are they healing their guts, they are paying attention to other parts of their lives, which can affect them more than other factors. As they feel better about themselves, they have more hope and optimism; they smile more and worry less.

These factors are not considered in most studies, yet they're important. Combined with the physical effects of better diets, the integrated effects of these factors—taking care of themselves, valuing their lives more, hoping for a better future—serve to improve health. Just like muscles work with bones and tendons in coordinated groups, changing misinformed habits for the better works in harmony with all other aspects of life.

THE BASICS: WHAT AND WHEN I EAT

My years of study and self-experimentation have resulted in a simple dietary practice that consists of a customized combination of natural ancestral eating that has been shown to be effective in research studies (see Resources). This way of eating is also most comfortable and effective for me.

My diet falls into these three programs:

- Calorie restriction (CR)—lower overall calorie intake than is "recommended" for my height and weight
- Low carbohydrate (LC)—very little, if any, carbohydrates from sources other than vegetables, and an abundance of high-quality unsaturated fat sources
- Intermittent fasting (IF)—regular, nightly mini-fasts of at least twelve hours, plus occasional reduced-calorie (only 800 per day) periods for three or four days

I eat mainly vegetables, salads, nuts and seeds, condiments, olive and other oils, as well as fish and meat as protein sources. I also take amino acid and plant-based protein supplements as well as vitamin supplements in case I'm not getting all the nutrients and phytonutrients I need from food. I pay attention to my gut bacteria and microbiome, knowing that the trillions of little critters and their balance affect my digestion a great deal. Sugar has never been a favorite of mine, although I will eat it when my daughters make something sweet. I've always liked cheese, which I try to limit.

My diet has become an uncomplicated routine in which the choice of *what* and *when* to eat is straightforward. Variety is not essential; I regularly eat the same foods because it's easy. Not obsessing about choice keeps me free from menu fatigue, affords me excellent nutrition, and gives me the bonus of lots of free time. My exceptions to this routine? Social occasions. That's when I partake in what's available without fussing. I concentrate instead on enjoying the company I'm with.

Similarly, our ancestors happily ate the same food every day. In their constant quest to eat, at least they had "something" every day. A need for variety may be a bigger problem for some than others. For many, my approach is radical and spartan. Most important, though, is eating only when I'm hungry and being willing to go for long periods with little or no food.

Here are the details of these programs and how they work together.

Calorie Restriction (CR)

Evidence mounts every day to support the same theory discovered in mice seventy-five years ago. (See Resources for studies cited.) Reducing calories or food intake without malnutrition occurring—and below levels previously thought were necessary for daily energy—not only extends life but increases energy and health. *How* this happens is still a mystery, but it probably revolves around challenging our bodies to become more efficient, operating on a lower amount of food than normal. Its essence is hidden in the complicated balancing system within all of us. A *Scientific American* article titled "The Exercise Paradox"[1] indicated there are calorie thresholds within our bodies. *That means increased energy output doesn't increase the number of calories burned beyond a certain level.* Thus, my body figures out how to maintain the same activity at a lower calorie burn or reduced calorie input. In some ways, our bodies become more efficient using only what's available. What a dynamic system!

Our models of "activity equals calories" are misconceived at best. In fact, Valter Longo states in *The Longevity Diet*[2] that stem cell production for new growth is *enhanced* by calorie restriction and fasting. This is especially important for staying healthy in our later years.

Calorie Restriction in Practice

How does calorie restriction (CR) work for me? I simply don't eat a lot, but at the same time, I make sure I'm getting the right amounts of vital micronutrients as well as macronutrients (fats, protein, and carbs). Remember, fatigue and lack of energy rarely result from hunger; our bodies can store enough fat to keep us going for weeks with no food.

I think we often use food as a convenient scapegoat for not looking at other factors affecting us—everything from inner emotional and spiritual stress to the quality of our mainly high-glycemic carbohydrate diets. Or is it possible we suffer from a lack of vital nutrients such as minerals and vitamins or not enough exercise and movement or even dehydration, boredom, stress, or many other sources of fatigue?

Like the detox I started with, getting used to a calorie-restricted diet takes a few days or even a few weeks. Yet once I did, the benefits far outweighed any pleasure I was sacrificing. In fact, I realized that most of the so-called "pleasures" of eating had emotional roots. I could replace thoughts of eating with caring for my health along with appreciating and enjoying the feeling of *not* being satiated.

Losing weight is a natural part of any CR practice. It's how our bodies start to become more efficient. As remarkably adaptive creatures, humans can function in many different locations and climates with various diets and circumstances. Just think of the extremes of Eskimo life compared with desert life, and the lifestyles and diets of each.

Humans have a beautifully efficient system of storing every ounce of excess energy ingested in the form of fat. We then access that fat when food is scarce, allowing us to get along without substantial food for days at a time.

When I embarked on a CR regime, I felt as if long dormant channels and practices were reawakened within me. My body felt increasingly comfortable. In prehistoric days, the ability to sustain feelings of hunger was a magnificent survival advantage—and a far cry from today's scheduled eating until we feel full.

A Fortress against Hunger

For me, the combination of CR and low-carb eating became a fortress against hunger, with my fat stores easily going into and out of storage as needed. This change reawakened my evolutionary fat storage and burning system, replacing the one-way system practiced in our glycemic, high-carb, and insulin-heavy world. As mentioned, I can now go for long periods of not eating and even fasting for a whole day with no discomfort or energy loss.

The hardest part is the emotional terrain that involves how, what, and why I eat and drink. Stuffing myself as a reward, eating sweets as a treat, and drinking a celebratory glass of wine are triggers *not* related to hunger. Because something *tastes* good doesn't mean it *is* good for me.

Pause before Feeling Full

On a family note, I encourage my daughters to practice an old Japanese custom called *hara hachi bu*. It's marked by a pause in eating when they are 80 percent full. Residents of one of the Blue Zones, Okinawa, credit this practice with much of their reduced calorie intake, their leanness, and their increased longevity. They know that any additional food consumed will lead to stuffing themselves and discomfort. Yes, the days of having to finish everything on our plates are over.

When a friend of mine went to a doctor and said, "When I eat late and go to bed on a full stomach, I don't sleep well," she prescribed an antacid for him. He could have saved himself time and money by listening to himself and quitting the practice of filling up at a late hour!

AUTHORITY ON AGING—AUBREY DE GREY

I recently watched a TED Talk featuring Aubrey de Grey, a leading authority on aging and longevity. This hard-core scientist pursues medical breakthroughs to combat aging. He stated he doesn't believe we can do much to combat aging from a lifestyle perspective *except* for calorie restriction—that it's the *only* method with enough scientific credibility to merit practicing. (I disagree with him on that, but I do agree that CR is a vital tool in the longevity toolbox.)

After de Grey's talk, an average-build American man stood up to ask a question. The man claimed he practiced a range of health-enhancing methods so he could live a long life. De Grey started his response with, "Not unless you lose that belly and some weight, you won't live long." When it comes to longevity, "skinny" matters. (De Grey is as skinny as a rail.) Most doctors know that overweight people rarely make it into the "longest living" category. This is not fat shaming; it's an honest recognition that being overweight, especially in later life, isn't only a *health* risk but a *life* risk. Our experience with COVID-19 and its high mortality rate in overweight people put an exclamation mark on this point.

EMPTINESS MATTERS

The Buddhists say that all enlightenment begins with emptiness. Feeling empty inside encompasses physical, emotional, and spiritual realms. As a source of new beginnings, it includes seeing reality in a new way. It also enhances curiosity while seeking new options or changed behavior. Learning to be patient with my emptiness has yielded me much.

For me, the emptiness I feel physically from practicing CR reflects this overall state. It doesn't pretend that constantly filling up with food, ideas, activities, money, excitement, or anything else leans toward meaning or happiness. Rather, emptiness contains all the energy needed to be reborn, come up with new ideas, and move forward.

LOW CARBOHYDRATE (CR)

About two years ago, I took a genetic test that confirmed something I've instinctively known all my life: I am overly intolerant of sugars and carbohydrates, especially processed ones including all flours, sugars, and manufactured snack, junk, and factory-made food.

By intolerant, I don't mean allergic. As good as a bowl of pasta tastes and feels in my mouth, it also brings up fond memories of eating my favorite spaghetti and meatballs as a child. Yet it has a deleterious effect on my digestive system, leaving me bloated, gassy, and uncomfortable. Pasta doesn't move through me as well as the vegetables, protein, seeds, and nuts that have become my staple foods. Much discomfort is due to gut yeast, which I partially control with oregano oil and/or a probiotic called Saccharomyces boulardii. Carbohydrates also leave me feeling lethargic because they take extra energy for me to digest.

Blood Type O and Prehistoric Life

Multiple detoxes and lots of study have been required for me to realize, admit, understand, and adapt to a relationship between my blood type and prehistoric life.

My blood type is O, which tells me my genes run back to hunter-gatherer days. That means my ancestors and I never made the transition to agricultural staples, wheat, and other grains. Those with type A, B, and AB blood have a greater ability to use these foods for fuel than type O people. These blood types initially signaled an adaptation to the new food sources. No wonder their appearance coincided with the emergence of agriculture about ten thousand years ago. Yet today, type Os still make up almost half of the world's population.

Our bodies have evolved to be able to store one to two months of reserve nourishment in the form of fat—our energy bank. By comparison, we only store about one day's worth of carbohydrates as glycogen in our muscles and livers. Which of these fuels has sustained humans for millions of years? Fat. And most of our regular low-level activity during the day is fueled by fat, not carbs. Unless they're needed for an immediate boost to restore that depleted fast-burning glycogen, carbs are first stored as fat and then processed as fuel.

Glycogen and sugar get used directly only during high-intensity activities or under stress that requires extra energy beyond 50 to 60 percent of our maximum heart rate. That's when it's hard to stay conversational while exercising. We're huffing and puffing or at least breathing heavily with an elevated heart rate—an activity level aimed for in CrossFit or high-energy interval training (HIIT). Knowing this, I *regard carbs as quick-burning gasoline while fats burn slowly like steadily burning coal.*

The Role of Fight or Flight

Our evolutionary ancestors arguably had more need for a fight-or-flight intensity in their dangerous lives than we do today. Yet their carbohydrates came only from plants, leaves, seeds and nuts, in-season fruit, and roots like cassava—all accompanied by fiber to slow sugar absorption. And fruits then were no sweeter than a carrot. Occasionally, honey was the ultimate sweet treat for them. Yet accessing the hive and surviving the bee stings were so fraught with danger, it's a testament to their bravery that they ate honey at all. Imagine a modern-day sweet tooth climbing a tree and enduring life-threatening stings just to get a candy bar instead of buying one at a local shop.

Our ancestral bodies were never meant to depend mainly on processed and sweetened carbs for nutrition. It is an adaptation that humans were forced to make, first from grains we grew and then in modern life. Some of us weathered that transition and can eat carbs without gaining weight or getting sick. But 60 percent of us still have the older genes and don't process carbs well and even natural grains, according to Jeff Volek and Stephen Phinney in *The Art and Science of Low Carbohydrate Living* (see Bibliography). The risks of eating too much processed, fiber-depleted, high-glycemic carbohydrates are elevated for all of us, no matter our blood type.

Man's Best Friend Diet

Evidence is bountiful that a low-carb, high plant-based fat diet is our best friend when it comes to lowering inflammation. It keeps our brains and nerves healthy and reduces symptoms and underlying causes of diabetes. It protects against the onset (or minimizes the effects) of many autoimmune diseases such as rheumatoid arthritis, multiple sclerosis (MS), psoriasis, and lupus.

Insulin resistance is a particularly nasty side effect of eating too much processed carbohydrate. Insulin is our body's natural defense against having too much sugar floating around in the bloodstream. That's because sugar at high levels is *toxic*, and it can cause severe side effects and even death. At lower levels, it causes inflammation of all sorts.

Insulin helps regulate sugar levels and limit any inflammation from causing further damage. Yet our sugar and processed carbohydrate consumption might exceed what our bodies can handle. When it does, the level of sugar in the blood required to trigger insulin goes up. It creates excess sugar floating around and becomes a low-level poison. As a result, excess inflammation can run rampant inside us, attacking our most vulnerable body parts.

I've also read about claims that high-carbohydrate diets contribute to Alzheimer's disease, and initial symptoms can be slowed by changing to a low-carb diet.[3] These are not "proven" claims any more than diet recommendations or food pyramids of the past have proven to contribute to good health. Rather, they are inklings of hunches, common sense, and experience making their way into the mainstream beside scientific and medical findings. In the case of Alzheimer's, for example, many psychological, emotional, spiritual, and placebo factors are involved that might be overlooked.

Payoff of the Low-Carb Diet

For me, the biggest payoff of a low-carb diet occurs in daily living. I experience massive digestive, outlook, and lifestyle benefits every day. My energy levels are smooth and don't fluctuate.

I needed to give my body a few weeks to adapt to a seriously lower carb and higher fat intake. This process sometimes involves the body's formation of ketones, an alternative fuel our bodies use in the absence of carbohydrates. Yet once my body did adapt, I realized that cravings for food disappeared and I could go longer without eating because my body burned fat more efficiently than before. The formula for adaptation (as well as the jaded history of high-carb promotion by government and the food industry) is contained in the bible of low-carb life: *The Art and Science of Low Carbohydrate Living* by Stephen Phinney and Jeff Volek. (See Selected Bibliography.)

These authors are my kind of researchers. They look behind the scenes at the history of flawed or outright manipulated studies on behalf of those who stood to gain from high carbohydrate consumption. They also incorporate human evolutionary history. Doesn't it make sense that the closer we can mimic our ancestral diet of natural and available foods, the better our bodies will function?

Myths about Carbs

The myths that pervade about low-carb diets are slowly but surely making their way into the mainstream and being exposed. Among them is that humans need carbs for energy and that sugar perks us up. *Wrong.* Another is that LDL cholesterol and other harmful blood lipids like triglycerides will rise if you eat more fats. *Wrong.* (The jury is still out on saturated fat. Sticking to unsaturated fats such as avocado, seeds and nuts, and olive oil is my lower-risk path. It does not, however, exclude *all* saturated fat, which is present in most fat sources on some level.)

Another myth is that high fat equals high weight. *Wrong.* There again, factory-made processed oils are a severe source of inflammation, particularly when combined with sugar. Avoiding anything processed is the solution. Ample evidence on all these issues refutes what has passed for common wisdom since the dawn of mass-produced food almost one hundred years ago. As Phinney and Volek document, the carb-based food industry has been bribing lawmakers for years to ban fats and increase carb consumption. In *Food Fix*, Dr. Mark Hyman showed that the food industry's bending of the truth continues in both overt and subtle ways.

Since I have adopted my low-carb eating plan, my weight has decreased, my LDL has decreased, and my energy levels have remained stable over time. This result directly refutes these three classic myths. Instead, carbs, and especially processed carbs, are the enemy of health for most of us. (I exclude low-starch vegetables and fruit in season when eaten whole, including their fiber.) And while this diet flies in the face of comfort eating and diets that suit modern lifestyles, it is our natural heritage—and an essential pillar of my practice.

INTERMITTENT FASTING (IF)

Three meals a day was never even an afterthought in the big picture of our history. Nature gave us an appetite that told us to "eat when you're hungry," which was most of the time. Our appetites also told us "don't eat when you're full," which probably also happened rarely. Even if our ancestors did overeat, they balanced it with long periods of digestion. Three meals a day has only been common since we began working at jobs for our subsistence—that is, from the beginning of agriculture and now in modern living. Today, eating has become regimented by social, economic, and emotional needs, not biological needs.

I've found eating on a schedule to be unnecessary except for when *not* to eat—fasting.

Fasting is a millennium-old practice for health and spiritual enhancement that gives our body time to clean itself and to rest, recover, and heal without expending energy on digestion. When combined with low-carb practices, the amount of time I could not eat became a world I'd never experienced before. I was using plentiful fat stores to fuel my energy.

DAILY MINI-FASTING

I regularly do a mini-fast by eating my light evening meal no later than six or seven o'clock. Then I don't eat again until midmorning or early afternoon the next day. This is a version of the twelve-hour fast I learned doing my detox.

In addition, I regularly fast for twenty-four hours or more, once a month or so, having only tea, water, and supplements, perhaps with a spoonful of yogurt to increase their absorption. I've become completely comfortable with that practice. I admit, though, social expectations as well as eating for comfort or boredom trigger occasional lapses in this routine.

I can exercise during my fasts and usually feel clearer and more energetic *not* eating than I would by eating constantly. The exception might be doing a hard workout that depletes my glycogen levels. Eating a small piece of dark chocolate fixes that quickly.

This combination—intermittent fasting (IF) with calorie restriction (CR) and low-carb (LC) eating—works well for me because it provides lots of stable, high-level energy.

THE LONGEVITY DIET

After I had adopted my three-part eating plan, the aforementioned book by Valter Longo came out called *The Longevity Diet*. A researcher and juventologist focused on the mechanism of aging, Longo showed in longhand what my body and more limited research were telling me in shorthand. The eye-opening results I experienced confirmed I was on the right path.

Longo's rigorously researched and documented prescription for longevity incorporated versions of everything I was doing: 1) eating fewer calories, 2) concentrating on plant-based carbs, fat, and protein (some occasional fish), and 3) daily mini-fasting plus once or twice a year a five-day *fasting-mimicking diet*. Its benefits enhance not only regular preventive health but assist in healing as well. In disease studies that include cardiovascular, metabolic, and cancer patients and those with dementia, this protocol improved the outcome of their medical treatments.[4]

EATING AND MODERN LIFE

As much as they support each other, IF and CR represent a radical departure from contemporary living. If my eating schedule were once again regulated by social and business concerns, this practice would be impossible to maintain.

In modern life, we've gotten so used to feeling full that we've forgotten what it feels like to be hungry! Eat, eat, eat! The message is everywhere. Even health advocates focus as much on cookbooks as anything else to keep readers engaged. The experience of cooking and eating, the diets, the fussiness and novelty, the fascination with new restaurants and cuisines, the social conversations, and on and on. This has become a ubiquitous way of life.

I'm not diminishing the importance of food or even the value of eating good food, which I enjoy as much as anyone. The social benefits of sharing meals can't be overlooked. Yet our entire ancestral existence was based on real hunger, necessity, solving problems, and confronting the dangers attendant with food. These challenges could be celebrated when faced and managed.

Our bodies evolved these two ways to survive hunger: ketosis and fat-burning adaptation. However, we rarely experience these today. People aren't even aware of how grateful we should be for our ease in obtaining what we eat. We are largely divorced from the entire process of growing, raising, processing, or gathering food. Instead, we shop for it and buy quantities that are often wasteful and unhealthy. Today, we can even have groceries delivered, so we don't get the benefit of moving while shopping and carrying them home.

By not eating much and not obsessing over choice, my lifestyle has become wonderfully simple. I have more time to do what I want to do—spend time with my daughters, and not only at mealtimes. This extra time, along with enhanced energy, supports a more active lifestyle than for most seventy-year-olds.

Unless you've been starving for days, needing food for immediate energy is a myth. Rather, eating is for comfort, habit, boredom, and the endless lists of other, often subconscious, prompts we use to justify almost constant eating. That said, I still eat out and enjoy social dining, but I do it less than before *and* I go more for the company than the connection with food.

SUPPLEMENTS AND MICRONUTRIENTS

Given the varietal range of organic food I eat, my body should have everything required to nourish me and/or synthesize what it needs to. However, as mentioned, modern agriculture and processing has dumbed down the nutrient value and range of our diets. Foods today simply are not as nutritious as the wild foods humans used to eat.

Consuming supplements can be a valuable aid in maintaining health, provided there is a reason for it. People also use supplements as a "just in case" insurance policy. However, we don't know enough about the micronutrients and synergies they create inside us, or what vital processes they might catalyze. And relying on supplements because they are broadly recommended is not only silly; it's a possible health risk and a waste of money. Supplements are *not* magic bullets for better health.

That said, there are a few supplements I can safely assume will be more needed as I get older than when I was younger, including CoQ10 and some antioxidants. Other than those, I use supplements based on need. That need is determined by blood testing, by studies showing a correlation between certain symptoms and certain supplements, or by a desire to experiment.

The Need for Supplements

What's the dirty little secret about supplements? Like nutrition, my body first must *need* supplements for them to be effective. For instance, taking supplements like calcium and vitamin D to strengthen bones is ineffective unless I'm tasking those bones with physical effort that causes them to need strengthening in the first place. Simply taking the supplements and asking them to trigger bone growth by magic won't happen; movement and strength components are essential.

Vitamins and supplements can be valuable tools in my body's ability to restore and maintain itself at optimum levels. Yet they need to be called for by a body that's healing, repairing, and renewing itself regularly—something accomplished with activity, challenges, and engagement in life. Just sitting around watching TV won't provoke a need for restoration!

The preferred route for obtaining vitamins and other micro or phytonutrients is from food, not pills. This truth is especially relevant with calorie restriction. My body can adjust to lower energy input, but it might not be as successful in restoring itself without all the biochemical catalysts needed to support my complex molecular biochemistry.

In summary, I base what supplements I take on my active lifestyle. Because the breaking down and rebuilding process is at the center of my physical life, I want to get the micronutrients I need to support these processes. Still, I keep their consumption to an absolute minimum. Usually, I take supplements every other day instead of every day as recommended. Mostly, I rely on a multivitamin and a nutrient-packed green juice for my daily doses.

NUTRITIONAL BLOOD TESTS

When I started my research, I took a comprehensive nutritional blood test showing my body's natural levels of all the essential vitamins, minerals, amino acids, fatty acids, and other markers involved in energy production and body metabolism. To prepare for the test, I eliminated all supplements for four days so my body's natural levels of these substances could be measured. That would help me determine whether I needed supplements or not.

One surprise came back—a low level of lipoic acid, which I'd never heard of before. Lipoic acid is an antioxidant and a vital component of the energy cycle. I started taking it then and have continued. All my other levels, except for vitamin B-1 (thiamin), were normal without having supplements in my system. I continue to take these tests occasionally (with and without a supplement "detox") to see if those levels remain within range or need adjusting.

GUT BACTERIA: MANAGING THE MICROBIOME

If you're serious about gut health, I recommend reading Jeffrey Leach's *Rewild*. In this book, he documents his own experience with the Hadza people of Tanzania, one of the last hunter-gatherer people. They live in an almost prehistoric way and eat in what we'd call dirty and unsanitary conditions. Yet they have exceptionally healthy and diverse colon bacteria compared to samples taken from modern people living today. This is partly due to their diet free of sugar and processed foods—modern "treats"—that kill off healthy bacteria and encourage "bad" organisms like yeast to grow. And it is partly due to their intimate contact with nature, with dirt and bacteria. This contact has given them a high level of resistance to common bugs that would make most of us sick. Scientists today are just beginning to address healthier levels of good bacteria that enhance digestion, elimination, and all sorts of other health factors.

An example of this intimate contact is eating the raw (or lightly cooked) stomach of a freshly killed animal after wiping it off with dirty hands. From my many trips to that region, I know the local people are more "naturally" resistant to parasitical stomach bugs than visitors who wash every leaf of lettuce and vegetable before eating it or take antibiotics at the first sign of discomfort. With local people being exposed to these bugs from an early age, their immune systems can render them harmless. The Hadza, like many indigenous people, have virtually no incidence of cancer, diabetes, or heart disease.

Technically, our entire digestive system is outside of us. Its linings are more like skin than other internal organs, providing a selective and protective barrier with a complicated system of entry that protects us as well as nourishes us. Our bodies treat the food we ingest with enzymes and chemicals to break it down for absorption and kill anything harmful. This inner/outer world is owned by bacteria, known as our microbiome, which assist in digestion. Yet our immune systems are simultaneously on guard for anything dangerous while allowing friendly bacteria to exist.

Any part of this process enters our bloodstream through a highly selective absorption process. The quality of our inner digestive lining is as critical to our dietary health as anything else. Like a digestive tag team, good bacteria and fiber are among the most effective ways to maintain that health.

We are learning more about our microbiomes every day. This includes our skin microbiome, with new research showing some skin cancer treatments can be enhanced by replenishing depleted exterior bacteria. New evidence points to a range of diseases linked to a poorly functioning gut. Other studies show that bacteria can synthesize at least some of the essential amino acids needed to produce protein, thereby possibly lessening the amount of protein needed to consume in food. This is how a cow can build muscle consuming only grass without eating a bit of protein. Rather, it gets its protein from the colonies of bacteria in its four stomachs as well as broken-down fiber in the grass and hay that the bacteria "eat" before being absorbed by the cow. (See Resources for sources of this information.)

USING PROBIOTICS

From Leach's book, *Rewild*, I learned that consuming probiotics regularly is not necessary to keep our gut bacteria flourishing. Another study said the variety of bacteria in a healthy gut is too great to replenish with store-bought versions. Short of a fecal transplant, what *is* necessary to support a healthy gut is lots of fiber, both soluble and insoluble. In addition to the fiber pushing and pulling nutrients through the body, fiber is the gut bacteria's preferred nourishment, which allows bacteria to thrive and multiply on their own. The result? Enhanced absorption in both intestines. So, I give my gut bacteria as much as possible of what *they* like to eat!

Those who take costly probiotic supplements often don't know that a few forkfuls of fermented sauerkraut or kimchi have more healthy organisms than the most powerful probiotic supplement. I avoid washing salad and other leaves if they're organically grown with no pesticides. Why? The good bacteria in sauerkraut or kimchi originally sat on the cabbage leaves used to prepare these foods. Bacteria had a good environment in which to grow and ferment the leaves, thereby forming an even healthier and populous environment for themselves.

Organic vegetables and lettuce grown without pesticides have lots of these bugs and dirt all over them, and they are good for us. As Leach wrote, the healthiest thing our children can do for their digestion is play in the dirt like Hadza children.

One study pointed to the integrated pathways through which gut bacteria affect us. It cited a fecal transplant given to healthy mice from mice bred to show signs of autism. The healthy mice then developed the same symptoms. What an unexplored pathway! This could prove to be another vital area of exploring our friendly bacteria going forward. (See Resources for sources of this information.)

PUTTING IT ALL TOGETHER: MY TYPICAL DAY OF FUEL

The following describes a typical day's eating for me, including what and when. Living this way for several years, I have maintained or improved my activity levels, fitness, muscle mass, and emotional and cognitive abilities. My digestion and elimination are comfortable and regular. My body could be called thrifty, well-tuned, efficient, or even radical. It has adapted to my routine and seems to prefer it. Hopefully, this practice will reduce my risk of serious disease as far as insight, instinct, belief, medical data, and research can guide me.

Morning

Contrary to touted dietary advice, my mornings are eating-free. Instead of food, ingesting a combination of supplements and teas make up my morning routine, with no loss in energy and a continuation of the detox process from the evening before. I start my day taking supplements and drinking a green juice called ProGreens.

Specifically, I take a multivitamin, some chlorella to enhance the fasting detox, and lipoic acid. Every other morning, I add Neuro-Mag, Cognitex, as well as carnosine and creatine. The carnosine and creatine are for muscle maintenance; the Neuro-Mag and Cognitex are for enhanced brain function. They are made up of high concentrations of either magnesium or plant extract. If I've had a big workout the day before and/or consumed little if any protein, I might take essential amino acid tablets. Usually, I take a few *before* a workout as well.

Added to this is a cup of hot Japanese sencha (for more antioxidants, but mainly I like the taste) with the juice of half a lemon to enhance my nightly detox. Then I usually drink a cup of Japanese macha tea with lemon. Whipped together with a frother, it's yummy and energizing (also slightly caffeinated). None of this breaks my fasting from the night before.

All my life I've been dogged by breakfast messages such as "You have to eat breakfast!" or "It's the most important meal of the day."

Both these statements, for me, are old wives' tales of major proportions. Throughout my life, every time I ate breakfast, particularly a high-carb breakfast, I would crave carbs for the rest of the day, and I'd feel bloated and lethargic. Truth be told, I wasn't hungry in the morning *unless* I was nursing a hangover.

The way I eat now represents the most comfortable, focused, and energetic routine I've ever started my mornings with. On the days I take further supplements (usually every two or three days), I ingest them either with a light dinner or with a spoonful of yogurt and/or a chia seed pudding (almond milk, chia seeds, cacao and/or cinnamon powder, and vanilla).

Additional supplements are CoQ10, astaxanthin, gamma E, omega-3 fish oil, DHEA, GLA, and a vitamin B complex. All are either antioxidants or supplements that have an evidence-based connection with improved longevity as well as healthy blood, heart, muscle, and brain maintenance.

Lunch

Usually my biggest meal of the day, lunch is sometimes my only real meal. I eat anywhere from noon until four p.m., thereby giving myself a daily fast of twelve to fifteen hours. This meal usually comes after movement. If I'm not exercising before afternoon, I might have a small snack in the morning. Lunch is frequently either a big salad, organic and unwashed, or fresh vegetables, sometimes cooked and sometimes raw with hummus. I buy these at a local farmer's market that has different kinds of salad leaves—sorrel, mustard, claytonia, rocket (arugula), purslane, and mizuna that are rarely found in supermarket salad offerings. I add fresh herbs like dill or parsley or coriander (cilantro) as well as broccoli, green beans, carrots, or mushrooms. It might be accompanied with pumpkin seeds, sunflower seeds, and flaxseeds. Then I cover my salad with a mixture of olive oil, raw apple cider vinegar, and Thai fish sauce.

I take in additional protein—salmon, canned mackerel, sardines, eggs, chicken, and occasionally beef. My vegetable sources include a pea protein supplement that I mix into a kale and avocado smoothie, hemp seeds, and different seeds and nuts.

I find that protein is a much-misunderstood subject. Of the twenty-three amino acids required to make the full range of protein we need, only eight are essential amino acids (EEAs)—that is, our bodies do not synthesize them and they need to be ingested. What we think of as "complete" protein sources—meat and fish—contain all eight amino acids while many vegetables and plant sources contain one or more. Beans, nuts, seeds, and even vegetables such as broccoli contain surprisingly high amounts, which are all we need when combined. A vegetarian diet that's varied enough is not low on protein in any form. A stunning example is shown in the Netflix documentary *The Game Changers*. In the movie, the world's strongest man and a host of athletes in sports ranging from martial arts to professional football improve their performance while being on vegan or vegetarian diets.

That being said, my activity levels and strength training (along with a natural tendency to lose muscle with age) demands taking in adequate amounts of protein. When I don't, my body takes longer to recover and my energy levels lessen.

Dinner and Snacks

Dinner, which I consume by six or seven p.m., is either a *smoothie* with avocado, kale and herbs, ginger, chili, almond milk, and pea protein or a *snack* of anything around. Usually, that's vegetables, nuts and seeds, or a piece of whatever I'm feeding my daughters that night. I nibble while cooking, which makes up extra that goes into the mix.

If I'm still hungry after lunch, I eat snacks up to seven p.m. My go-to snacks are seeds and nuts, Wakame seaweed, 90 percent cacao chocolate, chia seed pudding, a carrot or snap peas or green beans with hummus, even a spoonful of almond butter. I find these foods are tastier than conventional processed snacks.

INDIVIDUALLY SUITED DIETS

This routine suits me, yet I admit that my lifestyle and personality dovetail with it as well. It's an uncompromising routine *except* when I want to enjoy meals with others for business or social reasons. Freeing myself from this routine *in my own way* has been part of my health focus as well as my later life journey.

Changing one's diet to more natural and less processed fare can produce profound effects. I've seen this kind of eating dramatically improve health, outlook, and probably longevity as well. It has worked in every independent and honest study I've read. Modern life and institutions fail to do a good job supporting healing and preventing disease. Will that change anytime soon?

My own health started with a personal commitment, plus effort and study. Connecting with the source deep inside me, it began and remains an individual journey. Adequate and high-quality fuel is a basic necessity for that journey. Yet I have learned that most of my past beliefs were misinformed at best. As far as food goes, I like to keep it simple, keep it real, and keep it the way it was intended by the world that shaped us. When in doubt, I eat less and move more.

SUBTLE ASPECTS AND OTHER DIMENSIONS

We humans are born hungry—for nutrition, knowledge, experience, love, and a deep, genuine, self-realized, and wholehearted life.

I came with a wondrous program that this glorious universe endowed me. What I feel as hunger is more than the need for food; it's the totality of what I want and I need, the vast realm of actual and perceived needs inside me. My "real" needs are those I was born with and those I was programmed with—the basics nature gave me to survive and grow. Going without them will damage me in some way.

To the extent these early needs were understood and met by others strengthened the life-supporting and life-appreciating systems inside me. To the extent they were misunderstood or supplanted by non-genuine needs or beliefs, these systems became stunted or imbalanced. The way this plays out in later life differs in all of us. In my case, I've felt a deep hunger to recapture that early spirit. I want to learn how my emotional system of childhood suppression worked and then change it. Despite being buried under a mountain of false illusions and emotional baggage, this hunger never went away. Encountering my mortality in later life has made it all the more poignant.

In the chapters that follow, I examine the interplay of these factors on my health, activity, longevity, and quality of life that are vital for my well-being.

12

To Live Is to Move

"I don't exercise to get fit or be healthier; I do it to enjoy being alive."
—THICH NHAT HANH

"If it doesn't move, move it."
—KELLY STARRETT

My philosophy of movement mirrors what I believe about nutrition. For 99.99 percent of human history, living and moving were synonymous with the everyday reality of human life. We moved to hunt, forage, farm, protect, and defend. We also moved to find or create shelter as we interacted with others and marked celebrations. Unlike our ape cousins, our survival depended on almost constant movement, from running to dancing, to evolve as a species.

The recovery I experience from a workout—multiplied by 100,000 generations and countless days of struggle, survival, and reproduction—has made me what I am and given me my capabilities and personality. The movement that our ancestors used to survive became the evolutionary force that shaped my body. The coordinated, multidimensional motions of throwing, climbing, standing, walking, looking, running, squatting, pushing, pulling, reaching, and lifting sculpted my body, bones, and tissue. The need for these movements created myriad energy pathways in the form of nerves and circulatory systems. New challenges and capabilities that came with walking upright enhanced the independent use of my arms and hands as well as my mental powers.

These actions were performed in touch with the rugged, sustaining earth. No chairs and sofas existed; the earth was our floor, our garden of gravity, what we rested on and rose from, and what sustained us. We interacted with its rawness every minute of every day. Because of it, our bodies evolved with stronger legs than arms, feet and toes with abundant nerve endings, and flexibility, balance, strength, and speed. The movement we value today in sports is derived from our ancestral past.

For many, that history of movement exists no more. Their preoccupation with "comfort" has usurped a natural need to move. Sitting in a chair—a right once reserved for royalty—is commonplace today. To think otherwise seems foolish (unless you are Katy Bowman or Kelly Starrett, highly respected movement anatomy authorities who understand how harmful sitting has become for us). What passes for movement in our daily lives is a little walking or limited exercise in a gym.

None of this replicates the natural, harmonious, and integrated movement our bodies are capable of and what they need to be sustained. Until only a century ago, most people worked with their hands at physical jobs or at least stood most of the workday, which made them fitter than people tend to be today. No wonder we're experiencing an epidemic of conditions such as bad backs, low energy, frailty, and other diseases!

There is no truer adage than "use it or lose it"—especially as we get older.

THE JOY OF MOVING

I look forward to the joy of moving in all sorts of ways. By rediscovering myriad ways of living in my visceral body, I realize how much I'd been denying myself this basic life force and the pleasure it brings.

As expressed earlier, I had a negative opinion of my physical abilities as a child. This was reinforced by competitive team sports that the boys in my school were encouraged to pursue. Nonathletic boys weren't even encouraged to participate in sports and got picked last for teams. Outside of sports, other natural movements were either not available or frowned upon.

For the first time, when I went to summer camp from age eight to twelve, I began to appreciate the skills and movement our ancestors needed to survive. From crouching down to build a campfire to canoeing through wild river rapids to building a lean-to shelter from branches and leaves to shooting a bow and arrow, I viscerally remember connecting with the activities of our human heritage. I still love being surrounded by nature, using my skills on camping trips with my daughters, and walking in the woods or climbing hills.

BUILDING HOUSES

When I graduated from college, I shunned any white-collar career path I could have taken. Instead, I moved to northwest New Jersey and learned to build houses. As a framing carpenter, I used skills I had learned in our family cabinet-making business in Newark. Framing houses was extremely hard physical work, cutting and carrying lumber up ladders, banging nails, lifting, balancing, moving my body in every possible direction. I spent entire days, summer and winter, in the fresh air braving whatever weather conditions were thrown at us.

As a result, I became lean and muscular. With the full weight of accomplishment and fatigue at the end of each day, I felt great. This unconventional choice was one my mother couldn't get over for her college graduate son. Yet in those formative years, this lifestyle grounded me in many areas. Among other things, I learned the basics of motivating a small, well-coordinated construction crew, an experience that served me well during my printing career in my thirties, forties, and fifties.

Until that point, modern life had robbed me of robust physical activity, much to the detriment of my health, mobility, and spirit. Hard work became the entryway back into my body. And while I went back to a white-collar business career, I never forgot what it felt like to be fit and lean and energetic. Being apart from it felt like a separation from something vital, which is why I started swimming in my forties and took up yoga. But finding my way back into my visceral, somatic body took more than just an hour a day of exercise.

In chapter 4, I outlined the beginning of that journey. The book *Younger Next Year* initially outlined my early experimentation with moving again so I felt better, had more energy, was more muscular, and stayed lean. I read books and articles explaining the increased health benefits of movement. At some point, I found a deep connection inside me that tied together my movement, my evolutionary interests, and how I could sustain my health and mobility. I had good company in learning with Daniel Lieberman's *The Story of the Human Body*, Katie Bowman's *Move Your DNA*, Kelly Starrett's *Becoming a Supple Leopard* as well as *Deskbound*, and B.K.S. Iyengar's *Light on Yoga* and *Light on Life*. I read inspirational stories like Olga Kotelko's, who competed in sports actively into her midnineties, and trainers such as Ben Greenfield were helpful teachers too.

INTEGRATION

Beginning with the basics of aerobic exercise, yoga, and other strengthening and flexibility work, I slowly incorporated movement into my daily life. Trips to the gym supplemented my other activities. My yoga practice deepened dramatically. The mind/body/spirit connection brought subtle awareness to different parts of my body as I learned what they do and how they function.

The energy within and around us has myriad physical components, and we experience them in every part of us. Every second presents an opportunity to sit straighter, stand taller, walk better, flex and strengthen different muscle groups and joints, and practice balance and alignment. Movement and bodily awareness are not confined to studios or gyms; they are part of life. How I feel inside is affected by my posture or by simply breathing consciously. This awareness has become a 24/7 way of life complete with the mysteries and truths of a constant teacher—my body.

PUTTING IT ALL TOGETHER: MY TYPICAL DAY OF MOVEMENT

Following is how I spend a typical day, including ways I put in extra movement as a regular practice.

Morning Routine

Every morning after my waking-up breathing exercises, I do a basic set of all-over motions to enhance waking. It's as much a prayer and gratitude session as it is movement. I greet the day, drink tea, and feel grateful for the gift of life. This consists of 15-20-30 minutes of mostly floor work such as scorpion kicks, mule kicks, giant crosses, yoga twists, gentle yoga poses, deep squats, push-ups, downward and upward dog, leg work with yoga belts, twists, pushing and pulling, walking on all fours backward and forward like a chimp, and whatever else comes to mind. All these focus on my spine and limbs moving in a slow, coordinated, and highly aware way. No part of this movement is intense.

Whatever state of mind I wake up in, getting blood and energy moving through my body and brain as well as flushing joint and bodily viscosity out of my system makes me feel alive. Even on recovery days when my additional movement is walking and standing, my morning workout acts as the bare minimum required to pay homage to my physical well-being.

Discovering Better Ways

Finding better ways to move became fun the more I got over the age-old notion that comfort and ease are beneficial. These days, I stand more than I sit, particularly when I write. I take breaks regularly while working at my "standing desk" (i.e., the kitchen counter) and move around the house, picking up or using one of my many props. These consist of a yoga mat, yoga blocks, foam rollers, blankets and belts, a chinning bar, a light bar and slightly heavier weighted bar (5 kg), a Stick Mobility trainer, kettlebells (16 kg and 12 kg), a BOSU balance trainer, and a TRX belt system. These props add to my daily movement routine. And the movement itself often catalyzes new ideas.

Walking and Standing

When going out, walking is essential. I drive a car only in the summer when I'm in the country. If I can afford the time when I'm in London or New York, I forego taking the bus or subway for at least part of the way. If I do take either, I stand (not sit) and practice my alignment, balance, and yoga awareness. I can do isometrics and yoga anywhere, engaging certain muscles, standing up straighter, pulling or pushing the bars on the bus, or even just being aware of what's happening in my body. This approach actively engages my legs, hips, shoulders, neck, and head.

Feeling this subtle energy that goes beyond physical has been a huge benefit of learning yoga. Practiced correctly, it is relaxing and powerful at the same time—like my yoga retreat experience I described in chapter 9. Knowing that dysfunction and decline are caused by lack of circulation to one part of the body or another, I keep the blood and energy flowing, which can only be accomplished with movement and effort.

Rather than sitting, if I want to rest, I lie down or sit on the floor. I also occasionally collapse onto a sofa, but not for long. If I have to sit awhile such as in the theater or restaurant, I don't use the back of the chair. I stay conscious of my legs, hips, and shoulders supporting my upright back. This may sound distracting, but it becomes second nature with a bit of practice. As discussed in chapter 12, a collapsed, curved, or stooped spine brings more woe than just a stoop, for it can affect the heart, lungs, and other vital organs.

Moving More Every Day

It's a never-ending project to find ways to increase my movement and activity, particularly those that resemble what our ancestors did every day. So I carry groceries home in two heavy, balanced shopping bags. And I wear shoes that are zero-drop and minimalist—that is, no difference between heel and toe height to replicate barefoot walking. As I walk, my toes grip the bottom of the shoe, and I feel the ground almost directly, an action that originates in the upper leg if done properly. This gives my walk a slightly twisting torque that mimics natural walking and uses more body parts in unison.

Walking up and down stairways and escalators is an excellent movement generator. So is going barefoot indoors and most of the summer. I carry and lift suitcases and heavy objects as much as I can, even volunteering to help "older people." I squat down to get things out of a bottom cabinet or closet instead of bending over. Sitting on the floor allows me to get up and down many times a day, sometimes holding something heavy like a kettlebell. When properly aligned, my hips and legs stay strong and flexible, which in turn supports my balance.

Nature and Outdoor Time

I also strive to be outdoors in nature as much as possible. Yet I balance this by my love of cities—especially New York. When we spend summers on Long Island, the extra barefoot time in sand and on grass feels delightful. There, opportunities to move outdoors abound: gardening, boating, sailing, swimming, carrying, paddle boarding, and more. I even drag a 350-pound Hobie Cat up and down an inclined beach to and from the water, rather than use a roller—just to get the workout.

Most important, I get great satisfaction from doing all the activities an able, strong father does with and for his children, and I want that to continue for years.

Supplemental Practices
Yoga

The body awareness that's part of yoga infuses everything I do. It's the only practice in which the subtlety of inner body awareness mirrors the subtlety of how I experience life. The elements and sensations of it never cease to fascinate me.

With yoga, the practice that guides me to the inner gyroscope of my physical self, I sense space and the extra "hidden energy" that flows into a joint or a part of my body that wasn't evident before. I enjoy having the strength to hold a pose and work on it more deeply as well as the increased flexibility that happens when I use muscles, joints, and tendons in unison as nature intended and with fuller awareness. These inner signals also tell me if what I'm doing is or isn't effective.

One hidden part of the body is the fascia—a web of tissues that runs top to bottom and side to side. They aren't muscles; they aren't tendons; they're like a thick sheath around groups of muscles that keep the parts coordinated while moving. All natural movement relies on this coordination. Central to any good yoga practice (like the Iyengar style I do) is a deep awareness of this fascia network that corresponds to the energy meridians in yoga and acupuncture.

The Poses

Specific poses or *asanas* are less important than what energies I bring and how harmonic they are in relation to the rest of my being. The degree of articulation and engagement to do a pose properly requires a lifetime of study. Subtle energies are uncovered, awakened, and given new life. According to B.K.S. Iyengar himself, yoga ultimately is meant to bring us closer to God by getting closer to the core of ourselves and our miraculous body and spirit. Practiced fully and properly, yoga is far more than a fitness modality; it's a sacred study of life.

I practice a range of *asanas* both regularly and remedially. Standing poses include triangle pose, warrior pose, forward bend, and extended angle pose. Seated and supine poses include downward dog, upward dog, and fully engaged floor positions in which their difficulty belies their seeming simplicity. I practice different twists that benefit my joints and internal organs, getting blood flowing into places rarely addressed in modern life. Inversions include headstand, handstand, elbow stand, shoulder stand (both supported and not), as well as a special Iyengar-developed hanging rope inversion. Various balances and backbends round out the poses.

Once I was taught the basics, I found *Yoga, The Iyengar Way* to be a ready guide to all the poses. But I believe having a good teacher from the start is essential. I'm extremely grateful to mine, Nikki Costello, in countless ways.

Although there are myriad forms, motivations, and classes of yoga available today, I prefer my own simple yet deep, genuine, and sometimes difficult version. Nikki tweaks my poses from time to time, but generally I practice alone because I can concentrate better and not compare myself to others. This is my journey, after all.

I subject myself to a yearly trial involving yoga, which has become a feature in our household and one of Iyengar's tips for a long and healthy life (see tips in the Resources). *On my birthday, I do as many bridge poses (also called wheels or upward bows) as I am years old.* It's a moderately difficult pose; I face up with my feet and hands on the floor and my pelvis and back raised upward into an arch. Once there, I lower my head and touch it to the floor like an upside-down push-up. I started doing this when I was sixty-four years old and have maintained it every year, with seventy-three repetitions on my most recent birthday. My daughters love that I can still do this!

The Gym

I often go the gym where I can use props and equipment I don't have at home. It's also an environment of effort and is more social than doing everything on my own. Sometimes I learn something new from watching a trainer with another person. Mostly, I ignore the fashion set who show up to look good; their "body sculpting" vanity exercises don't interest me. Apart from some of the aerobic work, pumping iron and static, sagittal, one-plane exercise machines are meant to work muscles for appearance only. In my opinion, they don't replicate natural coordinated motion and aren't designed to benefit health. Besides, how I look in the mirror doesn't reflect how healthy I am.

Nonetheless, if I stay in my space and focus my awareness, the gym provides features I like.

Aerobics

During the Covid-19 lockdowns, I found ways to continue my aerobics training by walking, biking, and improvising high-intensity sessions. Yet I missed the gym and its wider range of options. It offers different forms of aerobic work with stretching afterward and includes high-intensity interval training (HIIT) roughly once a week. That's when I push myself as hard as I can, whether I'm on a stationary bike, a rower, an inclined treadmill, or the gym floor swinging kettlebells or doing floor exercises.

High-intensity work is a maximum exertion technique shown to be very effective in boosting aerobic power. Claims have been made that it increases stem cell production—the specialized, supercharged cells responsible for new growth and damage repair. (They are also the cells that take over in the womb and early growth to make us who we are, so you can see how important they are.) Other than competitive team sports like my Masters swim team featuring "wind sprints" as a regular part of training, this is one form of aerobics that hasn't gotten a lot of attention until recently. It replicates the fight-or-flight responses that our ancestors experienced regularly and involves short bursts—anywhere from ten to sixty seconds of maximum effort and heart rate above 85 percent of maximum followed by an equivalent or slightly longer rest period before the next burst.

I usually judge the number of reps doing this exercise by how exhausted I am. I do them until I'm huffing-and-puffing tired and can't do any more. And while each interval recovery is necessary to gear up for the next one, when I'm finished and exhausted, my recovery from the effort feels like a taste of paradise.

Although HIIT plays a largely overlooked part of health, it's a rhythm our bodies were primed for during most of our existence (like running from a lion). We experience almost none of that anymore in our modern lives. It's also a proven way to build endurance and stamina as I push my body to renew itself. Yet even at this level of effort, I would probably run faster if an actual lion were chasing me.

For me, the benefits to my heart, muscles, circulation, energy, and more outweigh the steady, monopaced aerobic activity I did previously. Yet I still do some aerobics at comfortable levels (like I started with from *Younger Next Year*) at a heart rate of 60 percent or so for enjoyment. I applaud anyone who starts there and progresses to higher levels of health. But for many, a putting-in-my-time syndrome includes one-hour distracted gym "fixes" they believe to be all they need. That's better than nothing, of course, but especially as we age, the amount of daily movement we need—and are capable of—is more than people realize.

ON TORQUE AND FASCIA AND NATURAL MOVEMENT

In the gym, I've learned to lift or pull weights using a full range of twisting and torque motion. Our bodies were built for a more complete range of movement than we use them for today. These movements involve the full breadth of every bodily system and a seemingly magically coordinated complement of muscles, bones, tendons, fascia, nerves, blood, and more. Moving one muscle at a time to "sculpt" it is *not* how we were intended to move. Only by becoming aware of how coordinated these movements are have I been learning to replicate that movement in exercise. The fascia wrapping these sets of muscles and tendon and bone are the pathways we're *meant* to move. (A good reference is *Anatomy Trains: Myofascial Meridians for Manual and Movement Therapists* by Thomas Myer.)

One example a trainer friend showed me is to use a weighted bar inserted into a swivel base called a land mine or dead man. Using two hands, I bring it up from the floor beside me while squatting and twisting. Then I stand and turn, lifting and raising the bar over my head. This motion uses entire sheaths of fascia from my feet to legs to shoulders to arms and all the muscles and joints in between. There are many variations when using this equipment; some involve jumping, stepping, and skipping.

Another exercise is a one-handed bicep pull on a TRX strap from a squatting to standing position. This includes a reach with my other arm at the top of the pull. The entire torque of my body, especially my hips and glutes, generates strength and not just my arm.

Using the full body as the source of maximum effort is how nature created us and how our ancestors moved for most of human existence. Variations of these exercises provide the natural, all-over, coordinated body motions I'm striving for. I do my best to mimic them in daily life such as lifting a suitcase into an overhead compartment and twisting at the same time, with my legs doing more of the effort than my back.

PURPOSEFUL INNER AWARENESS

Also included in movement is inner awareness, something I discovered from yoga. This is why I practice alone—to concentrate and *feel* what's going on inside. Our ancestors rarely moved without a purpose, even if it was simply the joy of moving. While they walked, they were looking for food, being ultra alert of everything around them, fully engaging their minds and hearts. Think back to the original marathon in ancient Greece. It was run to convey the important news that the Greeks had prevailed over the Persians in the Battle of Marathon. Its purpose was *not* to achieve an ego-driven personal best.

When exercising, I'm never on the phone and rarely listen to music. When I look around in the gym, I see most people want to "get it over with" as they divert their attention. Being disconnected from their bodies, they want to experience as little effort and discomfort as possible. I used to do this as well, knowing I would benefit in weight loss and appearance, yet not wanting to experience the process directly.

Today, the sheer pleasure of the workout, even the hard bits, provides sustenance for me. It's one way of entering those subtle inner pathways that reveal so much. That's why I usually have a notebook nearby and jot down new insights. It's yet another enjoyable benefit of moving.

SUBTLE ASPECTS AND OTHER DIMENSIONS

In *The Body Keeps the Score*, Bessel van der Kolk describes how different sorts of movements can awaken the body to "re-feel" not only the movement itself but any underlying emotions tied to past trauma. Movement isn't only about fitness and physical health; it's intricately linked to our emotional inner life. The subtle energies we experience in yoga and meditation can point directly to spirit, emotion, and substance. Feeling good after moving—whether it's dancing, fitness-oriented, or practices like yoga, Tai-chi, or Chi-gong—isn't only about endorphins. It involves caring for ourselves, connecting with a vital part of us, and reconnecting with age-old rhythms nature created for us.

One practice that's benefited me greatly is somatic experiencing (SE). It features spontaneously moving, with another person as a trusted witness, to see where movement takes me inside and out. The witness gets as much out of this practice as the mover, and then we switch roles. Through SE, I've been able to access emotions and images that have eluded me in conventional psychotherapy. Given that most of our evolutionary time was spent without language and thought, how we moved, looked, and acted formed the basis for communication. It's how we made our emotions known. (Chapter 12 on balance and posture deals with additional subtle factors that affect us in later life. I address them not only physically but as the sum total that has been an integral part of my practice.)

A LESSON FROM NATURE AND MY DAUGHTER

My daughter Jess loves animals, wants to be a vet, and avidly loves horses to the extent that she plays polo and works around stables. In our conversations about longevity and movement, she has told me things about horses I didn't know. For example, the average life span of a horse is twenty to thirty years. Depending on what they've done until that point, they get sluggish toward the end of their lives and don't want to do much except eat and hang around their stalls.

Polo ponies (called by that name at any age) are exceptions to this pattern. They need a daily running routine to keep fit for polo matches. Far and away, they lead more active lives than other horses. Throughout their life span, they run at all different speeds and stop and turn quickly. Because of their activeness, polo ponies live up to thirty-five years, with many still playing polo into their early thirties. Those extra five, ten, or fifteen years gained by moving more than other horses represent 15 to 40 percent of active, thriving, vital living. That teaches us a lot!

13

Balance, Alignment, and Posture

"Suppose we had no skeleton? Our whole being depends on this stiff, inflexible, in a way lifeless element in us. We do not carry it as a dead weight. It carries us."
—MARY MIDGLEY, *Beast and Man*

There is no more telling sign of aging than the classic hunched-over posture and shuffling or stiff walk of an older person. A host of factors bring on these conditions. They encompass the spectrum of mind, body, and spirit—factors including weak muscles, bones, and fascia; lack of life balance and self-image; and belief in the inevitability of aging. Such resignation leads to the heavy burden of carrying out life. It can result in conditions ranging from limited breathing capacity to inner organ compacting to frailty and poor balance marked by a general downward spiral in outlook and physical function.

THE SITTING-RISING TEST FOR BALANCE

A Brazilian doctor, Claudio Gil Araujo, developed an uncannily accurate predictor of near-term mortality called the sitting-rising test. You simply lower yourself to the floor, legs crossed, and then get up again. The aim is to do this without support. If you can do it smoothly without touching anything with your hands, you get a score of 10. Every time you touch something, including each attempt at raising yourself off the floor, you take a point off that number. If you wobble or don't move fluidly, you take a half point off that number.

Dr. Araujo followed people he gave this test to for years. Out of two thousand patients aged fifty-one to eighty, those with scores less than 8 were found to be twice as likely to die within the next six years. Those with scores less than 3 were five times as likely to die within six years. Overall, for each point less than 10, there was a 21 percent decrease in mortality. These results reveal that the combination of factors going into balance are good predictors of death, not to mention quality-of-life issues. Older people, after a serious fall, often rapidly decline due to frailty, dependence, and fear of falls happening again.

TOTALITY OF WHO WE ARE

My balance involves strength, awareness, special organs, muscle and tendon tone, sensual acuity, mental outlook, and emotional stability. Ultimately, my physical balance comes from gravity. It is the body's natural response, honed over billions of years, to this universal force affecting life on this planet. *Balance is harmony and synergy.*

I have an innate sense of balance that's not only physical but mental and spiritual—one that's essential to survival. When things get out of balance on any of these fronts, I feel challenged. Being in balance appeals to me because it feels harmonious and integral to life. The perfect balance of a tree growing upright is the combination of its strength and alignment in response to the gravity it constantly inter acts with.

How amazing that I seem to understand things easier when I feel balanced—whether it's in my body or something I'm perceiving like a work of art. My life gets out of balance when something isn't right. Certain physical aspects I can address with sense and movement. Other mental and emotional aspects can cause anything from high anxiety to mild stress. In addition, spiritual aspects relate to how I interact with the greater world around me. When I am balanced, I experience feeling at peace with myself and the universe—when everything seems to make sense. I also feel the sheer joy of being alive to experience this magic.

I used to take my physical balance for granted. Yet, nowhere else in the animal kingdom is the head balanced constantly on top of the spine. This core sense of balance is emphasized by our two-legged upright movement. Standing on two legs took apes and then humans millions of years to accomplish. In apes, standing is a short-term, ungainly way to aggressively grow tall, access certain foods, and frighten others. For humans, standing became a way to give us permanently increased height and full use of our arms and hands. Our species gained an entirely unique perspective on life and movement because of it.

Once an intimate, well-balanced connection between our feet and the ground was established, our fundamental existence changed forever. In the process, we lost the ability to live in trees, but the advantages of being on the ground with our new capabilities made the sacrifice worthwhile. Our bodies have changed in countless ways that contribute to who we are today.

My unique sense of balance is a product of all this—the first step of being human.

LESSONS FROM TREES

If a tree started growing on an angle, likely it either wouldn't live or would have to devote so much energy to keep from falling that its survival would be threatened. And unless its root system of support was overly strong, the tree would topple.

The same applies to us. If our spines begin to curve and go out of alignment, the pressures that build in other areas to support ourselves make for a radically altered and unbalanced system. The space needed to fill our lungs as well as what our internal organs need to maintain full circulation get reduced. We either develop overly strong muscles in one area and let others become weak, or we have chronic problems by leaning too much.

The same thing happens with too much fat, especially belly fat. Stresses and strains appear where they shouldn't. The body works too hard to maintain itself erect. Circulation decreases; blood vessels and nerves get pinched, including those in the heart. This further reduces overall health, creating pain and medical issues usually addressed by symptom relief. Once the imbalance begins, it's hard to locate where it started. On the process goes in a slow spiral of decreased strength, ability, and balance.

BALANCE AND THE SPINE

Balance starts with my feet touching the ground like the roots of a tree and works its way up my legs, spine, neck, and head. Staying balanced is my natural inclination, the path of least resistance. Good posture falls into place as long as I stay aware of my natural response to the ground and gravity; it's where gravity and balance encourage our bodies to be.

Most yoga practices emphasize the spine, the place where the body's core energy resides. The powerful energy that runs our biology exists in abundance throughout the spine. Many posture and balance issues can be addressed by paying attention to what the spine is doing and how it's being supported. Advanced yoga practitioners even use the chakra system of the spine, where primal energy is stored at the base and can be encouraged to rise to the top of the head in gradual, refined ways. As we awaken this energy and encourage it to move up our spine, it becomes more and more subtle as it flows through the stages of the spine, the belly, the heart, the throat, and the head.

Poor posture, like slouching, drastically affects this energy and our biologic as well as our psychic well-being. Energy can be compromised in many ways; *the most basic is not being aware of what good posture is.* Many who have lost that connection try to alleviate a back or neck problem without examining *what supports the back and neck* in the first place.

I have noticed one symptom that signals a gradual immobility later on. It's a stiff or frozen sacroiliac joint at the base of the spine. The person walks in a way that the hips don't move freely one leg at a time; they begin to walk in a waddle, the entire hip moving at the same time. Once people walk like this, it doesn't take long before their overall mobility and balance suffer. The source of these "stiff hips" is lack of strength in the muscles supporting the hips, glutes, hamstrings, and all other supporting muscles in that area. Once weakened, overall circulation to the entire area becomes compromised. That result begins with stiffness and usually develops into a host of other problems.

Hamstrings and glutes, the strongest muscles in the human body, are vital to standing up and walking on two legs. They are, in turn, supported by an intricate system of lesser muscles, tendons, nerves, and fascia that also need to stay strong and flexible. Modern life presents many shortcuts for not using them, from sitting too much to slouching on sofas to lack of movement and other "comforts" in general. To be restored to their full vitality, they need extra strengthening and movement. Not coincidentally, it's the area most affected by "bad backs," which lead to more doctor visits and workdays missed than any other reason. Symptom relief for these has spawned a major industry—from orthopedic surgery to pain relief to chiropractors and osteopaths. Yet, for the most part, bad backs are preventable or curable with knowledge and effort. (See my tale of healing in chapter 21, in the section "Learning to Walk Again.")

THE EXPANSION OF BALANCE

One time, I was doing a tree pose in yoga, balancing on one leg and placing the bottom of the opposite foot on the inside of the balancing thigh. As I usually do, I focused on my breathing and a spot on the wall. Yet, I was also aware of all the muscles, bones, organs, and other parts of my body at work holding the pose.

Recognizing the seamlessness and harmony with which my body enabled me to stand this way led to further noticing the same integration I was experiencing with the forces around me—among them gravity, the air I was breathing, and the air that was touching and supporting me. I felt as if the entire universe was supporting this effort, inside and outside, all interrelated and harmonious. Like power, it first felt like an otherworldly force—effort and no effort all at once—coming from the outside as well as the inside. Yet, this is how the universe works. I've experienced this more expansive sense of balance ever since.

Nothing functions on its own. Where there's a push, there's a pull.

Where there's an effort, there's a reaction. Where there's strength, there's flexibility. Where there's an inhale, there's an exhale. Recognizing this complicated quality of my existence in even the simplest things has enhanced the wonder of my daily life and pervades my physical, mental, and spiritual world.

INNER STABILITY

I use the term "balance" for more than standing up straight. It also refers to a sense of inner stability, a harmonious place inside. More accurately, it's when I feel that the challenges in life and my ability to meet them are appropriately matched and I can work toward achieving them. The integration this sense of balance has on my physical body is largely unexplored territory in today's world of medicine and health, yet it fascinates me. *And it feels right.*

All of nature shares a respiration cycle: effort and rest, effort and rest. My body is wired to this rhythm; it's how I define my days. I work and then recover, I eat and then digest, I read and then ponder. To the extent of always being "on"—exerting myself like I used to, fueled by caffeine, sugar, alcohol, and toward goals out of balance with my inner life—I lost this primal balance I'm now regaining. Upsetting this rhythm can be as harmful to my well-being as any bad habit.

A damaging aspect of balance is being disconnected from nature. We think modern schedules and pursuits are valid replacements for awareness, rhythms, and contact with nature. We don't know where that tipping point is, but once we get out of balance, we see a decline. David Suzuki called this "sacred balance" in his book by the same name. As a society, perhaps we have already passed the tipping point regarding how we treat nature and our fundamental disregard for its power over our lives. To the extent we believe we can control nature and set ourselves apart from it, we are misinformed at the very least.

INNER BALANCE AND HEALTH

A basic sense of balance lies at the center of my life as a visceral quality like a hunch or a gut feeling or a guide. Discomfort, imbalance, or a sense that something isn't right can feel like the absence of feng shui in a room. Most important, I'm learning to trust and appreciate my sense of balance as a visceral emotion that guides my practice as well as my life. Although often bumpy, I'm realizing balance was not something I had to learn. Rather, it's part of the inner guidance system I was born with. Knowing I have a need generates imbalance; getting that need satisfied reestablishes it. In my case, it's like a keen awareness that things are not right.

I've learned to get into balance by adjusting to changing conditions while developing new tools and understanding along the way. I'm reminded of two books by Kelly McGonigal on stress. In her first book *The Willpower Instinct*, she writes about the harm stress does to us and ways to control it. Yet, as she studied the subject further, her ideas evolved, and she wrote her second book, *The Upside of Stress: Why Stress Is Good for You, and How to Get Good at It*. In this book, she points out the importance of stress in our lives as a way of learning to overcome it.

I believe the stress we feel (including the imbalance and sensing things aren't right) is the catalyst we must deal with so we can grow. *Realizing stress* and then *dealing with it* is finding a way out of it—the age-old, hard wired way of coping with hardship. In my physical body, non-chronic inflammation serves the same purpose. It is the catalyst for healing.

Our current preoccupation with comfort, ease, and pain relief reflects the modern belief that life should always be balanced and easy. Even worse is wanting to be seen as "not affected" by stress while hiding the emotions that come with it. Thus, we believe if things are not effort-free, then something is wrong—or *something is wrong with us*. What a surefire way to keep stress circulating!

We feel this imbalance on many levels. As stated earlier, recovery after exercise is how my body grows slightly stronger as it finds a new equilibrium in reaction to the effort. On a deeper level, my train ride epiphany was a recognition of a basic imbalance and the need to find a new center. This process has taken many years, yet the results of following my instincts since then have been lifesaving. My efforts reflect the endless work of the human condition—one I hope to have many more years to perfect.

INTERCONNECTION

I sense a subtle link between these two forces: 1) the balance and harmony in nature and the world around us and 2) the physical balance and alignment I feel and the emotional balance inside me. This interplay underpins the way my personal universe operates. My body is constantly being shaped while being subjected to gravity and fully integrated with my heart, mind, organs, nerves, blood vessels, bones, and muscles. A kind of supreme balance governs all the interplay within me and outside me. Yet balance is also found in constant movement, even when my experience of it is stillness and stability. It all operates as a system. Fiddle with one aspect of the balance and things get unsteady due to always trying to find a new equilibrium. If the equilibrium is lost for too long, the system decays and eventually collapses on itself.

Viewing health from this standpoint is a revelation that doesn't only apply to posture and standing balance. In the gym, I see people who concentrate on one aspect of their fitness such as muscle building or aerobics. They do the same movements over and over, mistakenly thinking this is how they will best benefit. As a result, they can run or lift, but as they get older, they can't bend over or balance on one leg.

For me, health and activity are tied to a well-rounded, multifaceted system of balance. As dancers know, seemingly effortless balance depends on their entire body being strong, flexible, and mobile.

PRACTICING BALANCE

Fostering balance in all these respects is at the core of everything I practice. This does not mean standing straight like a soldier or being emotionally rigid, stubborn, or habitually intolerant of anything new. On the contrary, it means staying flexible, strong, aware, accepting, and open. I find that staying balanced *physically* enhances my ability to stay balanced *emotionally* and *spiritually*. When done in harmony, they complement and catalyze each other. When any of these is forced or overdone, my system gets out of whack until I find my center again. This imperfect process requires experimenting all the time because the quest for one's center and sense of inner balance is always present.

By making balance and alignment part of your daily awareness, you can come up with multiple ways to practice. Lift up one leg and balance on the other to feel how subtle and complex it can be. You can try getting dressed and undressed while standing on one leg or the other, including putting on shoes and socks. That helps you see how balancing engages all your senses, muscles, bones, tendons, as well as your awareness.

THE GIFT OF YOGA

Yoga is at the heart of my physical balance practices. Inversion poses such as headstands, handstands, shoulder stands, and elbow stands are obvious ways to balance. So are one-legged stands like the tree pose. Yet even simple postures like standing can be transformative if I concentrate on body parts that are stuck or need space and I determine where my effort goes as I lean in one direction or another. Once I learned the subtle sense of aligning one bone on top of the other, gravity began working on joints and other body parts just as they were when I first learned to stand. Even walking becomes a different experience when I become aware of my balance and how my body parts are coordinating to make me move. Cultivating this awareness requires concentration, but it's well worth the effort.

A WALKING MEDITATION

The form of walking meditation that has been advocated by Thich Nhat Hanh integrates the entire body and mind with balance and movement. It calls for walking slowly, step by step, feet shoulder width apart, and carefully placing one foot in front of another while concentrating on breathing and what the body is doing.

Years ago, I learned a version of this called *cloud walk*, in which each step is taken very slowly as my weight shifts gradually from one foot to another. I balance solely on my main leg before taking the next step. I note the essence and complexity of how the body balances with each step. This kind of balance and centering lies at the heart of many Asian martial art and exercise forms such as Tai Chi and Chi Gong. They focus on breathing and awareness as well as slow, deliberate, and balanced movement.

BARE BONES

Our bones don't support themselves; they are supported by a system of muscles and tendons that, in turn, make up a mutual dance of effort. Keeping these muscles strong so the bones align the way they should is essential to good posture, continued bone strength, and bone growth. Any movement that pushes, pulls, or twists benefits bones and joints as well as muscles.

Again, gym exercises usually do little in this regard. Natural movement does a much better job. One physiotherapist who works with older people suggests putting weights in a backpack when walking around, saying, "Joints need effort to strengthen and survive."

I urge anyone with postural problems to work on aligning the spine sooner than later. It's easier tackling this in your forties and fifties than later in life. Alignment requires unlearning bad habits, relearning new ones, and freeing up chronically inflamed joints and other tissue. The result is a fundamental sense of alignment and joint flexibility that benefits not only one's capacity for movement but how you generally experience life. It doesn't come without effort, but the human body can get there with practice and an awareness that's present every day.

14

Recovery, Repair, and Renewal

"For every thirty minutes of practice, rest for five minutes."
—BKS IYENGAR

"The wisdom of stopping and healing is still alive in animals, but we human beings have lost the capacity to rest."
—THICH NHAT HANH

In my forties, I swam on a Masters swim team at our local pool. The coach, who was once affiliated with an Olympic team, worked us hard. On average, we swam about 15,000 yards (eight-and-a-half miles) a week, including two supervised workouts of drills and sprints. I had never trained so hard in my life. I had also never competed at that level. We had regular regional meets with other Masters teams, and I was in races with other swimmers in my five-year age bracket category, which at the time was forty-five to fifty.

During training, I always felt tired, but the fatigue temporarily wore off once I got back into the pool and started moving again. However, the days I took off each weekend gave me nowhere near enough time to fully recover. And I was always hungry.

I had never heard of tapering.

TAPERING

Six weeks from our first meet after roughly four solid months of training, our coach announced the beginning of our taper. The workout that night would be 80 percent of our usual one. She also gave us a guideline for reducing yardage every week until the meet. The final week was to be no more than five hundred yards of easy swimming a day, just to stay loose and limber. The purpose of the taper? We could reach full recovery and maximum strengthening to let our bodies do what they do naturally when subjected to stress—that is, heal and get stronger.

All the hard work we'd done for months had built up a level of expectation in our bodies that resulted in faster times when we raced at the meet. Various forms of tapering are tried-and-true training methods in most competitive sports, particularly swimming and track. Times at meets tend to be faster than during training, partly because of encouraging this maximum recovery.

Tapering is not merely recovery; it doesn't just restore what was there before. Healing makes us stronger and encourages *renewal*, which is a better version of what existed before. And here lies the ultimate lesson—the miracle that exists within each of us. Nature has given us this great gift of health. *Our bodies get better and stronger with use, provided we challenge ourselves enough and allow enough time and energy to recover.*

This healing is our most potent ally in a quest for longevity and quality of life. And whether it comes from exercise and diet or renewal from emotional trauma and stress, our body and soul are endowed with this miraculous ability to heal and get strong.

A BENEVOLENT ALLY—RECOVERY

I realized I hadn't paid enough attention to this vital phase of health—recovery. I'd always veered toward staying moving and keeping working, thus violating natural rhythms. In my case, whether it was a grin-and-bear-it attitude toward resting or an "I deserve a reward" attitude by overeating or overdrinking, I didn't let recovery and healing have its time and space. Yet, since my health journey began, I have given recovery more time, attention, and gratitude. This benevolent force inside, hidden for much of my life, protects me. Having its energy in my corner has been profound, not only in my physical health but also in my inner life.

Nothing to Do, Nowhere to Go is a dog-eared book I've been reading and rereading for years about the teachings of an eighth-century Zen monk named Master Linji. It is edited and commented upon by Thich Nhat Hanh. Its message always inspires me, no matter when I pick it up or where I turn to. In teaching his students the essence of Zen Buddhism, Master Linji tells them to just be themselves and appreciate who they are.

This is the miracle of Buddhism and of life—right here and right now—and full of wonder. Students will never learn it by rushing around and filling their lives with prescribed studies or by spending their days being *perceived* as being someone as opposed to *being* someone.

ENCOURAGING RENEWAL

As I became more familiar with how this energy of healing pervades my existence, I learned about encouraging it in my life. It's what I felt on the train ride and in my first detox in all its physical, mental, emotional, and spiritual dimensions. This energy can't be harnessed or controlled, but it can be understood and encouraged. It has its own rhythms and timetable. I use the watchwords harmony, synergy, and benevolence to encourage its existence.

Staying aware of something is the surest way to get better at it, a process that happens seemingly automatically. The often invisible marvel behind making progress on anything goes on in the deep recesses of my psyche. I can't take credit for my mind always pondering, but I can appreciate and allow it. When I do, I am benevolent to myself as well as the world around me, letting both express themselves naturally.

Yet renewal can also be inhibited when something inside, either conscious or unconscious, denies its power. I can also prevent renewal when I don't give it time and freedom to do its work or I don't feel deserving of receiving its benefits.

MY IMMUNE SYSTEM AND ITS RHYTHMS

As noted earlier, my immune system is at the heart of healing. The never-ending work of maintenance and recovery inside involves the complex biochemistry of cellular respiration and housekeeping. Under normal circumstances, not only can each cell in my body stay healthy, but it *knows* if it's healthy or not. When a cell senses something is wrong, it tries to repair itself. And when it cannot repair itself effectively, it's programmed to kill itself and be replaced by a new, healthier cell.

As I get older, this process, called *senescence*, doesn't work as well as it did when I was younger. My job is to keep it functioning well for as long as possible.

Everyone's body has these two phases or rhythms: sympathetic and parasympathetic. They exist balanced, side by side, in everything we do. My heart beats and rests, my lungs inhale and exhale, I eat and digest, I move during the day and sleep at night. The parasympathetic phase, the resting part, fosters rebuilding and renewal, yet it needs the stimulus of the sympathetic part. A rough balance between the two keeps the whole system humming and at maximum potential. An out-of-balance system where one phase predominates becomes fertile soil for dysfunction or illness. My immune system depends on balance to function well.

The same goes for emotional issues. When too much anxiety and stress is not balanced by periods of restoration and healing, my body experiences chronic, continuous inflammation. It never has the chance to heal; it's always on the alert for danger. Fixing emotional issues is different and more subtle than fixing relatively straightforward physical ones. Yet resolving emotional issues by discovering their underlying truth is as important to my well-being as any physical measure. In fact, the emotional and physical sides are complementary when I practice integrated healing.

The most effective ways to heal are related to issues described in Part I. Healing involves the less active parts of nutrition (digestion) and movement (rest) or an enhanced version of emotional and spiritual healing. Through them, I'm trying to harmonize my inner life with the rhythms of evolution and the natural world. For example, allowing the seemingly static phase of digestion is as important as the kind of food I eat. Similarly, exercise is only the catalyst for strengthening my body. The real work happens *after* the effort as well as *during* it. They go hand in hand, like yin and yang.

This is the rhythm of nature for getting better—a never-ending two-step dance the universe has been doing since the beginning of time.

HOW I RECOVER

I used to take the recovery phase for granted, ignoring it or impeding it by drinking and/or overeating. I had a hard time slowing down and giving recovery its time and space. Unless I was severely sick or sidelined with an injury, I put my endless to-do list front and center. Even now, my preferred recovery routines involve some activity such as pondering. But I also allow complete idleness because I've learned how productive and inspirational it can be. That's when new ideas, memories, emotions, and insights can transform the way I view my circumstances and make a difference.

Contrary to modern practices, the surest way to overwhelm the digestive system is to eat a giant meal and then sit around without moving. Studies have linked insulin spikes and inflammation to this fairly common practice. As Jared Diamond points out in *The World Until Yesterday*, our ancestors almost never overate and usually moved or danced at feast and celebration times. Paying reverence to *all* sources of life, including food, was what these gatherings celebrated, but food wasn't the center of the occasion.

The best way to digest and stay active is to avoid eating too much in one sitting and then moving easily, walking or at least standing, for a short time afterward. Collapsing on the sofa can be tempting, but I feel its effects in low energy and digestive discomfort. As stated earlier, my preferred inner state, physically and mentally, is an "aware emptiness"—not the bloated feeling I'd get by filling up. When I have overeaten, getting back to feeling less full combines moving (usually a walk or other gentle activity) and deep breathing. These increase the blood flow to my gut to boost my digestive energy.

As far as what to eat during recovery, I don't change anything from my normal pattern. If I have done a hard strength workout, I might make sure I'm getting enough protein to provide the building blocks for new tissue being created. Yet I usually get enough essential amino acids floating around my system from my regular diet to accomplish this. (Of the twenty-three amino acids needed for complete protein, only *eight* of them are not manufactured by the body and must be ingested. Meat and fish, some pulses, and some nuts contain all eight. Most vegetables contain one or more proteins and can provide complete amounts if my diet is varied enough. In a pinch, I supplement with an essential amino acid product.)

I add to this my continued practice of fasting and intermittent fasting, both of which are recovery and healing practices of the highest order. They allow my system to fully digest as well as fix itself. Most of this work takes place while I sleep, the vital center of all of nature's renewal efforts.

The Miracle of Sleep

In *Why We Sleep*, Matthew Walker gives a thorough treatment of not only the benefits of sleep but also how modern life limits our ability to receive those benefits. In the first chapter, he writes:

> Two thirds of adults throughout all developed nations fail to obtain the recommended eight hours of nightly sleep . . . I doubt you are surprised by this fact, but you may be surprised by the consequences. Routinely sleeping less than six or seven hours a night demolishes your immune system, more than doubling your risk of cancer. Insufficient sleep is a key lifestyle factor in determining whether or not you will develop Alzheimer's disease. Inadequate sleep—even moderate reductions for just one week—disrupts blood sugar levels so profoundly that you would be classified as pre-diabetic. Short sleeping increases the likelihood of your coronary arteries becoming blocked and brittle, setting you on a path

toward cardiovascular disease, stroke, and congestive heart failure . . . sleep disruption further contributes to all major psychiatric conditions, including depression, anxiety, and suicidality.[1]

Walker makes a bold claim that appreciating how powerful sleep is and getting enough would transform society, slow us down, and help us be more thoughtful, considerate, and ultimately healthier. While I agree with his ideas, I would go even further to say the psychic and spiritual benefits of sleep are as important as the scientific and medical ones.

During sleep, all conscious activity is shut down, a vital period that every living organism shares on some level. Nature runs the show by its own rules. Sleep involves everything I was born with as expressed by my DNA and life experience. My physical as well as psychic life is healed, restored, sorted, and cleaned. My conscious mind plays no role here. Rather, nature functions at its most natural—*the full power of an eons-old system running through every cell of my body.*

What happens while I sleep? Healing tops the list. I allow my body to do what it does best for as much uninterrupted time as it needs. To this end, I go to sleep around nine p.m. For some reason, I've developed a pattern of waking up in the middle of the night for an hour or so after four to six hours of sleep. I use this time to breathe, meditate, ponder, and sometimes worry before falling back to sleep for two to four hours. In Matthew Walker's book, I was comforted to read about two distinct phases of sleep. The first is a total shutdown of mental activity, a deep restoration of the body. The second is when we dream and sort through mental and emotional issues in addition to physical restoration. My pattern of sleep seems to mirror this rhythm.

Sleep is pure autonomic nervous activity run by the hardwired operating system nature has taken billions of years to give us. It's the vital key to restoring and strengthening our body's systems and organs. Other than allowing time for and appreciating sleep, I have no conscious control over it.

The endless miracle of sleep restores and renews, heals and strengthens every aspect of my being, especially when I've put in an effort that encourages healing. When I wake up in the morning, I feel plugged directly into the fundamental power of the universe working its mysterious magic on all aspects of my body, mind, and soul. Somehow it knows exactly what is needed, and the more I harmonize with its rhythm, the more I can enlist its power.

When I feel stuck on something, have difficulty writing, or face a tough issue, I ask the power of sleep to help me. Before going to bed, I say a prayer asking for light to be shed on the problem. I pray to the universal power of healing contained in the deep mysteries of my body and brain. It doesn't always deliver in ways I expect and can take more than one night. But most of the time, this prayer approach works. I wake up in the morning with a new way of viewing or even clues to resolving a problem. What a deep, mysterious ally to have at my service.

My Cues for Healing

Sleep works best when my conscious mind is not being controlled or interfered with. Its natural, deep healing ability is eons old, an infinitely complex process of housekeeping and growth that scientists are just beginning to understand.

Like our environment and all of nature, my body recovers best when left alone to do its built-in work. Allowing my body to work naturally and using my senses, instincts, and a few breathing techniques are almost all I need to *feel* how recovered I am. I use only one modern diagnostic, heart rate variability (HRV), which is explained below.

Surrender and self-benevolence as well as faith and reverence for the power of renewal become powerful allies—and not only for my physical body. I'm discovering how the pathways to health are intertwined. When I sleep, nature isn't limited to healing only one aspect at a time; all of me is recovering—mental and spiritual as well as physical. Thus, recovery efforts can be aimed at any one of these realms and sometimes fostered by inputs from another realm. For example, I have experienced relief from anxiety by doing subtle movement or deep breathing. Likewise, my physical symptoms recede by acknowledging the underlying emotions, usually anger, causing them. The subtle realms of interconnection inside form an endless journey of discovery. (See Part III, which features examples of how this integrated process has helped me heal from mental and physical problems.)

When Problems Surface

Before reviewing my regular recovery regime and special modes I use in my waking life, let me address an important element of my regimen. When a serious symptom occurs, I resort to *all* available means of diagnosis and treatment to figure out the source issue. Yes, medical diagnosis is an essential element but not the only one.

A good example involved a set of symptoms centered in my solar plexus and stomach. I felt bloated and uncomfortable. The center of my rib cage felt tight. Symptoms came and went, and my energy levels remained good. I thought the cause was something digestive, but my recovery didn't respond to changing or limiting my diet or taking additional probiotics to clear up any imbalance. Curiously, my symptoms got worse the day after a big workout. Although this didn't keep me from doing my usual routine, it created discomfort. Over time, I decided to look more closely into the issue.

I first sought advice from a medical doctor, then I went to a psychotherapist, a somatic experience teacher, and a personal trainer, in that order. I trusted all four from prior experience. After I described the symptoms, we worked on possible causes—from diet to my training movements to slow breathing meant to relax, reintegrate, and recirculate blood flow to the affected area. I was also free-associating on the feeling itself.

The results were revelatory. I discovered that I hold a great deal of emotional tension in my solar plexus and stomach, possibly caused by a multitude of physical and mental triggers. Even the medical doctor said my physical issues were probably connected to something emotional, as many digestive symptoms are. Relief came from working on relaxing my abdomen by breathing and concentrating on the feeling and where it would guide me. My symptoms haven't disappeared entirely, but the experience has evolved into a kind of early warning signal. Either something is amiss inside, or it is a signal to stop, reflect, and take time to recover.

I've learned that when a sizeable emotional insight makes its way to the surface—something my unconscious thinks I'm ready to handle—it makes its presence known via different kinds of anxiety. I used to try and relieve the tension with distractions like entertainment or alcohol or even resorting to pain relievers. I've since learned that when I can *tolerate* the discomfort, which can include physical symptoms that last several days, my subconscious presents itself in the form of a new insight or understanding. This process is not easy. However, I am getting better at it. Still, I'm so used to creating a diversion that this kind of awareness doesn't always get a chance to work. Instead, it goes back down the rabbit hole to stay hidden in my subconscious.

Yet when I *can* tolerate the discomfort, it greatly aids my inner healing. *Discomfort and anxiety are voices from the universe telling me to "pay attention!"* This happens in all realms: physical, mental, and spiritual. Yet, when I've allowed anxiety to surface, I've received positive feedback in the form of new ideas, emotions, insights, solutions, inspiration, improvement, and relief. That makes tolerating the discomfort easier.

Importance of Time to Recover

Modern life can deprive us of natural movement and naturally sourced food. We can also allow it to deprive us of time to recover. By packing our days with endless activities, we avoid the simple yet awesome experience of simply being alive. Even vacations are filled with itineraries, exotic destinations, tours, places to visit, and food to eat. Simply "being" is regarded as a guilty pleasure.

I used to think that being busy was the only way I could feel important—even more important than those other people racing around doing the same thing. (I always saw myself as *much* busier and *more* hassled than them!) My challenge today is to accept the grace and quality that comes with idleness. Not surprisingly, the most important new insights seem to spring from nowhere at these times. I also find peace and quiet and appreciation regularly—both in everyday life and even in doing mundane tasks. I once was able to find new insights only on a tranquil beach "away from it all."

Many modern training techniques give advice on ways to shorten recovery time. Various supplements or electrical stimulation devices claim to make recovery happen more quickly. Some even claim to shorten recovery time from a hangover. I've tried a few of these "hacks"—schemes that invite the "do-ism" of modern life to supersede natural rhythms. Yet nature has been healing us for eons; it's the real master of renewal. Other than keeping myself well-nourished while recovering, which includes having enough protein to rebuild new tissue, I let nature take its course, guided by my senses. Keeping in touch with the subtlety of my body and being—and paying attention to my distinct inner rhythms—works better than following a prescriptive course.

The Heart Rate Variability Tool

However, one contemporary diagnostic tool I use faithfully dovetails with my recovery philosophy—heart rate variability (HRV). HRV measures the health of the autonomic nervous system (ANS), the part that functions in the background to maintain overall health. Heart rhythm is an enormously complex phenomena made up of inputs from every aspect of our being: brain, heart, emotion, activity, breathing, and so on. Our heart rate increases slightly as we inhale and decreases as we exhale. HRV measures how "varied" that difference is. The inhale is the active, sympathetic phase, and the exhale is the resting, parasympathetic phase. HRV, then, represents a snapshot of the underlying ANS and how well-tuned and balanced these two phases are. The higher the HRV, the more recovered we can be. High HRV also indicates more resiliency to stress and more flexibility.

By comparison, low HRV has been linked to symptoms from depression to cardiovascular disease to anxiety to a shorter life span. This data has become a fairly accurate predictor of heart attacks. How? Low HRV indicates if the body's systems are in a stage of alert, trying to fight whatever is wrong. High HRV is linked to better health and longevity, not to mention a higher quality and less rigid way of life. *It indicates that no significant problems exist for the body to react to.* Illness and anxiety aside, for me, the day after a heavy workout usually results in a lower HRV, but after a day of low-level activity and recovery, my HRV bounces back to a higher state.

I take my HRV measure most mornings before I get out of bed, using a finger pulse reader and an app from Elite HRV. Sometimes the result fools me, pointing to a higher or lower level than how I feel. It has become a regular part of my diagnostic tool kit. (See other toolbox contents in chapter 16: Metrics, Diagnosis, and Support.)

Circulation Is Always a Friend

Although it's hard to resist, probably the worst thing we can do to recover from exertion is collapse on a sofa. *Recovery depends on blood actively circulating through the muscles, organs, and brains to eliminate toxins and rebuild.* This doesn't mean we should not rest. Yet I find staying active or at least engaging other areas of my body usually enhances recovery.

To rest, I either stand up or sit on the floor, not in a chair or on a sofa because these postures aren't conducive to good circulation. Keeping in contact with the ground has benefits often overlooked, among them not staying in one position too long. Our ancestors had three basic positions to rest: standing, sitting on the ground, and lying down (or sleeping). Standing and sitting on the ground shaped our bodies; that's what they were built for.

Yet, modern life has conditioned us to use chairs and couches, the softer the better. In *Move Your DNA*, Katy Bowman illustrates more than forty ways to sit on the ground or floor. The hard surface, shifting, and getting up and down from a low level keep the muscles and blood moving to enhance the recovery process. It also keeps my legs stronger and improves circulation.

Using chairs and sofas as a substitute for the floor is one of the biggest causes of movement problems in later years. Realize that chair sitting, especially nonconscious slouchy chair sitting, negatively affects recovery, posture, strength, and flexibility.

ACTIVE RECOVERY AND RESTORATION

Standing and walking are other ways of gently moving while recovering. I write standing up and usually move or shift my weight back and forth while doing so. In addition to enhancing my recovery, I'm practicing balance and posture. Staying conscious of my posture fosters inspired thinking by keeping energy flowing to all parts of my body. I'm usually barefoot and wear loose clothing so I can stretch while I work. Sometimes all the elements of my being working to put words on the paper (or the screen) feels like a dance. At times when I'm stuck, I do something physical like take a walk to distract my conscious brain. Lifting or swinging a kettlebell and/or doing a squat or pull-up can work wonders on getting a stuck imagination unstuck.

Many yoga postures are specifically used for the purpose of deep restoration. The poses are restful yet engaging while enhancing circulation and energy in areas that need it. They range from simple sitting and lying postures to inversions and enhanced breathing techniques known as *pranayama*. Practicing these poses sometimes leads to meditation, sometimes not.

When I practice yoga for movement, an excellent source of postures is described in *Yoga, The Iyengar Way* by Silva, Mira, and Shyam

Mehta. It has full explanations for each pose and a cross-sectioned guide for which poses suit what physical and mental conditions.

Puttering and Physical Labor

I find puttering around the house and garden wonderful ways to recover actively, especially when I can self-benevolently practice doing nothing. I have always loved working with my hands, fixing and building things, gardening and all forms of physical movement, many of which mimic ancestral movement. I sense a kind of intense concentration and balance between mental and physical attributes through physical labor. It's not too taxing, and it affords me quality recovery time.

Writing

While not taxing physically, writing can take a great deal of effort. It is, however, my "sacred space," a term coined by Joseph Campbell that illuminates the new world I've begun to occupy.

Writing comes to me in many forms. The type most conducive to recovery is the simplest yet sometimes most illuminating—that is, the Natalie Goldberg–inspired practice of simply writing down what comes up inside. This form of free association uncovers threads from the subterranean reaches of my subconscious. It is also my source for poems and short stories. (More aspects of writing follow in chapter 15: Clarity, Grace, Wisdom, and Serenity.)

Deep Breathing

Deep breathing is an excellent way to recover *and* a productive way to spend time and encourage inspiration. Deep, slow breaths start with the abdomen and then fill through the back and the top of the lungs, stopping for a second or two at both the top of the breath and the bottom. Deep breathing engages with what is happening inside, allowing me to relax, especially on the exhale. This mirrors the body's own "relax" mechanism on every exhale, the "letting go" hallmark of the parasympathetic nervous system.

While we may regard letting go as doing nothing, the practice is in fact resting our overactive conscious minds and allowing the natural forces underneath to do their job. Knowing this process goes on in the background makes my life easier. I can appreciate the wonder that the 90 percent of me I'm *not* aware of operates on its own—to keep me productive and inspired, active and healthy. *That subconscious part is doing what it has been for billions of years on its own timetable and to its own rhythm.*

In addition to *pranayama*, other breathing techniques can enhance recovery and promote health. Many of them are outlined in the book *Breath* by James Nestor, who also addresses the physiology of breathing in general.

A favorite method I practice routinely is the Wim Hof technique. It consists of taking thirty to forty deep breaths and conscious exhales, then holding my breath exhaled with my lungs empty for as long as possible, then taking one deep inhale and holding it for another ten or fifteen seconds before a final relaxing exhale. I repeat this procedure three or four times. It feels wonderful! But more than that, it stimulates the autonomic nervous system and immune system to release hormones that encourage relaxation and boost immune function.

As counterintuitive as it might sound, deep breathing is based on lowering the percentage of oxygen (O_2) in the blood while increasing the percentage of carbon dioxide (CO_2). This encourages the cells to allow more oxygen into them. Measured with a pulse oximeter, I regularly see my temporary blood oxygen levels in the 70th and 80th percentiles while doing the breath holding. This tells me the method of breathing stresses my system slightly and temporarily to produce a recovery effect. My blood oxygen percentage bounces back to the high 90s almost immediately with the added kick of a recovery stimulated by the temporary stress.

Praying

Although the topic of prayer belongs to chapter 15, its role in recovery is substantial. Many times I feel stuck, either from fatigue or from something that's happened with my daughters or a friend or from a piece of writing or more. I might have overreacted in anger or impatience to someone and can't let it go. I might have had an encounter that dug its claws into me and won't go away. Or I might not like myself for a myriad of reasons.

A feeling inside tells me, "There's something to learn here. Stay with it, even if it feels uncomfortable. Don't dismiss or rationalize it." I'm not sure whether to take action and, if so, what it would be. Or I'm simply in a blind alley, stuck. When this occurs, the best response is to do nothing except *pray* for a resolution—simply let the forces of the universe inside and outside me do their work. This is also recovery, and it's as important as any physical recovery.

I'm only partially aware of what I'm praying to, for the powers I call on are more vast than I can ever know. Mostly, I'm praying to the power of life, of existence, of forces that allow us to enjoy all its wonders around us—any part of the mysterious world I don't and can't control. Yet it exerts a significant effect on my life.

Even if I perceive the problem to be *outside* myself, the only real solution is to find a new way to engage with it from *inside*. Prayer helps!

The Rhythm of Life

Where do I begin solving a problem or issue or stress with a person? With my attitude toward it. Sometimes this requires new insight about myself or a different way of viewing a problem or releasing an old belief and moving into a new one. Many times, an emotional pattern from my childhood has emerged from the depths and stepped in to seize priority. It makes its presence known from a place I can only fathom by emotions and association.

Prayer is my catalyst to engage that process, the grease to get the wheels to move and recognize that I have a problem. I find it particularly effective when I blame myself for the problem to begin with, as prayer alleviates my tendency to blame myself. And it often makes me feel better. Even while *I'm* not doing anything, at least *something* is being done to fix things through prayer.

Prayer firmly acknowledges I'm not in charge—that a force bigger than me is. Buddha himself woke up when he stopped trying and allowed the universe to guide him. I feel relief and surrender simply knowing I'm part of something bigger than myself. Again, much of what happens is, was, and always will be out of my control. But this does not mean my instincts and desires aren't valid and can't be acted upon.

Yet, I'm learning to dance with a subtle balance and rhythm. Trusting in an ultimate solution has been an illuminating path, even when that solution isn't always in line with my initial expectation.

WHAT THE RECOVERY PROCESS LIKES

To the extent that recovery, repair, and renewal form the centerpiece of natural existence, they flourish best under conditions that include space, time, freedom, nature, and unconditionality. The process also likes wonder, awe, and synergy; it dislikes being judged.

If I'm blaming myself for not doing well on my last workout, for example, my recovery from it will probably be impaired. Instead, if I go with the flow and take it in stride by doing other gentle, life-enhancing activities that are enjoyable—or even just doing nothing—my recovery will probably be enhanced.

Do I have any scientific proof of this? No. Does it feel right instinctually and do I believe it? Yes, even if it's a placebo, it does the job for me. Still, there's probably more to it than belief. Maybe one day, we'll understand the process better.

RECOVERY DURING SUMMERTIME

I've always felt deeply attached to the summer season when we keep our family's schedules as open-ended as possible. We spend as much time as warm weather allows in a rented house on Long Island. And we fill our summers with lots of active recovery, providing a wonderful respite for body and soul. Our days are lazy, unstructured, spontaneous, and surrounded by sea and fresh air. But it doesn't mean we don't do anything—sailing, paddleboarding, kayaking, fishing, boating, swimming, gardening, DIY, and eating joyfully take up our time.

My writing comes and goes in the summer, sometimes full on and sometimes in the background. In some ways, it's like revisiting my own childhood in a setup similar to being near a lake in northwest New Jersey. I have precious memories of summertime and want my daughters to experience its joy too. But mostly, I want to imprint the experience of deep recovery in their bones. Plus, we love spending time together and appreciating each other.

15

Clarity, Grace, Wisdom, and Serenity

*"My god, I have finally got it after eighty years . . .
The world is there in both modes.
It is not that the world changes, it's your consciousness."*
—JOSEPH CAMPBELL

*"If you change the way you look at things,
the things you look at will change."*
—WAYNE DYER

Benjamin Franklin called it Powerful Goodness. Jesus called it the Father and the Holy Spirit. Mohammed called it Allah. Buddha called it Nirvana. Lao Tsu called it Tao. The Hindus call it Atman. The Jews call it Yahweh. Some scientists call it the God particle or the God Force. Robert Pirsig calls it Quality. I call it the Great Guide or Power of the Universe or Life Spirit or Healing. Many call it God. Joseph Campbell has documented the many other names that this spirit of eternal being has been called throughout history in his four-volume series *The Masks of God*, as well as his other books.

"God" is the ultimate source and way of the universe, of nature, and of our being, and the wonderful visceral feeling we have when we connect with its harmony and synergy.

Whatever this eternal spirit is, its energy, power, and life-enhancing ways keep me healthy and alive. It courses through my veins, my thoughts, my emotions. It *is* me, and I *am* it. It is the ultimate source of inspiration and renewal—clarity, grace, wisdom, serenity, energy, beauty, illumination, strength, and more. It is also fatigue, being stuck, self-criticism, decay, and death. Its ways are an eternal encyclopedia of wisdom to uncover—the ultimate guide of life. And just like the single-celled embryonic me contained everything necessary for life, my entire being is a singular expression of the entire cosmos. The best way I know of keeping myself healthy in all respects is *cultivating and harmonizing with this spirit* as much as possible. In *Reflections on the Art of Living*, Joseph Campbell sums this up beautifully:

The goal of life is to make your heartbeat match the beat of the universe, to match your nature with Nature.

The more I practice, the more I find health to be an interwoven journey of body and soul. Ninety percent or more of each of us is the realm of dreams, emotion, and inspiration as well as the world of biological balance and regulation. It's where these biochemical and electrical systems meet in the tapestry of that inner world. And despite ample evidence of the role the subconscious plays on our health, people readily shun dealing with the world of how we feel and how it affects us.

However, I'm not willing to forego paying attention to this synergy. From what I witness and experience daily, the risks of ignoring or even diminishing the effect of my inner life on my health are too great. I have benefitted greatly from being aware of this interconnection on every level. If nothing else, I am a magnificent machine created by the universe. The unity of all my parts is paramount. To that end, fostering my mental and spiritual health as I travel on my longevity journey is as important as any blood test.

PASSION AND CURIOSITY

Spirituality is the direction that called the loudest, that became a passion ever since my journey on the train ride. Once I engaged the force of healing, the universe began to answer me, opening a path that was life-enhancing in more ways than my physical health. Experiencing the immediate "nowness" that comes with letting in this power surpasses everything I've ever known—the joy of having a moment capture the eternal, here and now.

As the world inside me changes, the world around me does as well. I'm no longer frightened of what I don't know. My experience deepens and, at the same time, becomes simpler and more complex. An apparent contradiction, yet these two qualities now coexist harmoniously within me. Learning new or previously hidden information, the digestive process of the mind has become a never-ending steady inner diet. Curiosity, awe, overcoming challenges, and getting unstuck have led me to more stepping-stones on the everlasting road of fulfillment and knowledge.

We are each a vehicle the universe has created to know ourselves and the world around us. Our flesh, minds, and spirits are joined in that calling.

ANCIENT RHYTHMS PRACTICE

The core of this practice has been around for millennia. I call it *ancient rhythms practice*, handed down as wisdom from seekers before me and on whose shoulders my knowledge squarely balances. My practices of yoga, meditation, breathing, reading, writing, movement, recovery, and balance help me make sense of what humans are all about. I spend time in nature and strive to see the universal underpinnings of existence. I practice "nothing to do, nowhere to go" as I seek to experience that minute wonder of existence.

Subtle energies make their way to the surface of my awareness all the time. This inner journey is not necessarily personal and private, yet it tends to be solitary. I'm seeking internally for answers and inspiration to harmonize with my external observations. I'm after the connective energy that flows between me and the world as I stay open to this awareness. My journey is a full-time occupation.

THE PLACE FOR WRITING

Most of my writing is not the free associative, recovery-oriented writing mentioned earlier. It involves writing this book, short stories, poems, and articles for my website at www.RonKastner.com. Once I get going, writing takes on its own life and leads me to new places—an endless inner journey to new lands where one step leads to another.

For me, writing is almost always spontaneous, and if it doesn't feel spontaneous after working for a while, I find something else to do that day. Where new threads come from are as deep a mystery as knowing where life comes from—an ever-present reminder of the powers of renewal and creation.

Writing likes a regular schedule. As writer Somerset Maugham once said, "I write only when inspiration strikes. Fortunately, it strikes every morning at nine o'clock sharp." My writing lasts anywhere from one to four hours a day. Like waves in the ocean, a rhythm of active and passive phases gives time to rest and renew, preparing for the next round of effort. Many prompts tell me when I'm out of gas or resist going further—its own dance of inner resolve and inspiration.

Yet inspiration also has its own schedule. I carry a notebook and/or the note-taking app on my phone and jot notes as new ideas come up. Many never see the light of day, but I've learned that writing them down and rejecting them later is better than forgetting them and wishing I hadn't.

PSYCHOTHERAPY AS A TOOL OF SELF-DISCOVERY

One area ancient practice doesn't cover specifically is psychotherapy or therapy, although some evidence exists. I consider it the only valid, modern add-on to the practices already mentioned. In the right spirit and context, psychotherapy provides an essential tool of self-discovery, combining evolution, the precarious nature of being human, the search for love, and the monumental role the subconscious and autonomic system play in our lives. It also gives me clues as to why I behave the way I do, inevitably leading to greater inner freedom as I uncover hidden dynamics stemming from my childhood.

Experiencing real change in my old patterns moves me toward solid ground. I incorporate the strong dynamics buried under the surface for years by remembering old feelings, then accepting the emotions and re-feeling them to reintegrate them. This process also provides the basis for allowing new, spontaneous behavior not dictated by previous patterns.

Like all of us, I was programmed to blindly follow and attach to my immediate protectors, my parents, for the first years of my life. For me, this attachment didn't go well, and my own nature and inclinations were overridden. I was forced into a pattern of parental protection that depended on *their* needs, not mine, to the point of associating love and care with those patterns. To survive, I forced my feelings into the background. Yet those feelings still exist, and the work of therapy is to reengage them. Healing requires moving away from any false definitions of love and care so I can rediscover my genuine needs. While I have been pursuing this practice for much of my life, my inner work in recent years combined with my physical health practice have proven to be the most productive by far.

Therapy also lends a hand in diagnosing and fixing physical ailments by integrating my body and biology. John Sarno and others including Alice Miller, Caroline Myss, Bessel van der Kolk, Gabor Mate, and Louise Hay have pointed to uncovering repressed feelings as a way to treat pain and ailments—with dramatic results. I believe that every physical aspect of our being has some connection to our inner world, sometimes direct and self-evident and other times subtle and needing to be unearthed. To this extent, I view therapy as a valuable aspect of any health journey, especially in my later years.

WHEN CLARITY IS NEEDED

My search for clarity is not some grand monumental quest. I usually experience results in everyday life. I will describe a major episode of how this works, one that made my inner and outer life easier to navigate. Here's what happened.

At one point, I was close to finishing writing this section as well as this entire book. I had set a deadline of before leaving for summer vacation on Long Island. Part I was complete and edited; I told my editor I would finish Part II in about two weeks and Part III in four or five. I eagerly set about rescheduling everything around this work except activities with my daughters. I devoted mornings and most afternoons to writing, which was more than I was used to. Feeling exhausted at the end of each day, I slept well.

But after a while, I lacked energy, and the writing wasn't flowing as it had been. Potential culprits were diet and exercise—too much or too little of either—or lack of *quality* sleep. Yet nothing seemed out of the ordinary. What I was writing about didn't seem to be the issue either.

I pondered, "Am I working too much and drying myself out?" But the schedule I had imposed drove me to keep plugging away. I had pushed myself before many times, overriding any inclination to take it easy, which had been a hallmark of my career and one I'd taken pride in. Through sheer endurance, the extra effort had often paid off.

One morning about six days into this deadline push, I didn't feel like working. Every pore of me screamed to give it a break. Yet I heard a voice inside say, "I HAVE to finish!" I felt like if I didn't do what I had set out to do, I'd fail. Caught between the two, I felt miserable and didn't know what to do. Then something changed in the form of these two words: "I want." I thought about how eager I had been when I began the book; I had *wanted* to finish it. But somewhere along the way, I had substituted *have to* for *want to* and imposed a new set of expectations. Deep inside, a "dictatorship of the should," as psychiatrist Karen Horney called it, had imposed itself. I became a victim of the "dictator's" plans to the point that the quality of work mattered less than my schedule.

When I could recenter the effort within my visceral self and create a palpable feeling of "I *want* to do this" and not "I *have* to do this," all the tension and fatigue disappeared. Replacing them was a sense of feeling grounded and even joyful. I was able to express my wants without feeling subjected to outside influences or a rigid plan. I ended up finishing the writing slightly later than planned, but the result was better, more genuine.

Time and time again, my journey has reflected this kind of experience—uncovering and working through false assumptions that had inhabited my previous life. I let my real self out into the light.

A CURVED HORIZON

For decades, I lived in that world of supposed certainty and truth—one of numbers, straight lines, fitting things together, being on time, planning, and avoiding mistakes, mixed with worry, control, and impatience. These faculties served me well in my life of achievement and recognition that had become so much a part of me, I couldn't escape them if I wanted to.

Yet I'm learning about other previously ignored faculties such as release, patience, gentleness, care, compassion, connection, and valuable poetic qualities that deliver more quality of life than my old one ever did. Because they're visceral and emotional, I feel these qualities deeply. They help me make decisions based on their full impact rather than only the rational part. They are the stuff of gut and conscience, of flesh and blood, in which my rational part works harmoniously with my newly strengthened soul. *It's what I experience when I step back and see that the straight line in front of me is part of a curved horizon.* Enhancing and exploring these aspects has brought me this new clarity and grace.

A SOLITARY PATH OR NOT?

I have chosen a more unconventional and solitary path in these measures than would be comfortable for most. Yet, a universal part of this journey is available for those willing to set out on their own singular path, if practiced honestly. Success can't be achieved by following another's footsteps. Joseph Campbell repeatedly points out how the great myths of history survived in our psyches—the hero's journey—by people forging their own path and entering the forest where no one had tread before, then pursuing what lay in waiting. The goal of this pursuit, the grail, represents an ever-deepening experience of what it means to be alive. It reveals where real truth and knowledge lie.

As Heinrich Zimmer once said, "You can't borrow God." Yes, you have to find your own version of God within the confines of your being. In a famous passage from Herman Hesse's *Siddhartha*, Siddhartha told the Buddha that, while he respected his teachings, he needed to find his own path just as the Buddha experienced his own enlightenment journey alone. When the Zen masters say, "Kill the Buddha," they mean *find your own way through your own being.*

Certainly, you'll find others in the forest around you pursuing their own journeys. It helps to know they exist—that the calling to take such a path is universal. We learn from each other in a camaraderie that's more about harmony than dependence. However, we ultimately need to face the struggle to achieve self-realization alone.

THE SPLENDID INTENSITY OF DAILY LIFE

One day I was doing laundry at a communal laundry machine at our summer rental house. I had lugged two heavy baskets of laundry and detergent fifty yards from our house when my older daughter, Jess, passed me on her way to the beach with a friend. Without thinking, I said to her, "You know, most of this stuff is yours and Lollie's. You could at least give me a hand."

Then in a flash, something clicked inside. Before she could reply, I quickly said, "Only kidding. I genuinely *like* doing this. It helps keep me strong and active." We smiled in recognition of something mutually okay, and she went on her way without feeling bad about not helping. In the moment after the first words came out of my mouth, I realized *this* was what I was living for—*making it possible for my daughter to enjoy her life because of having a fully functional older parent*. I recognized my initial words had been aimed at a guilt trip—just like those my mother said to me as a child.

I genuinely appreciated my ability to carry these two heavy baskets with ease—to bend down, squat, hang clothes on the line, reach, sort, fold, and use varied movements. After all, I was outside on a warm day. Every pore of my body took in the beauty—from the leaves on the trees in the wind to the surf lapping up on the beach. Our dog Lola joyfully followed me around. And I thought, "This is great. This is it—these moments of purpose and sheer joy. The harmony between them defines life. I'm so lucky, so grateful."

AHA MOMENTS

Treasured aha moments like this happen as an integral part of what I mean when I say, "I'm looking for clarity, grace, wisdom, and serenity." These elements have become a near-constant presence in all the forms of my practice, whether it's moving, eating, writing, or just living. They're *not* the product of achievement, accomplishment, recognition, or self-importance. I hear no trumpets blaring or angels singing. These aha moments simply heighten my overwhelming sense of integration, both within me and with the world around me. Usually unexpected and spontaneous, they can happen on a hot crowded subway or while I'm doing dishes, and they bring much inspiration and sweetness into my life.

Over the past fifteen or so years, I have made myself a more hospitable place for the ahas to visit. The grace I experience in these moments becomes a guide for how I can live and practice.

16

Metrics, Diagnosis, and Support

"The future of medicine is in YOUR hands."

—DR. ERIC TOPOL

The array of choices for diagnosing and treating ourselves can overwhelm us. If you define health the way I do—integrating emotional and spiritual factors with the physical—the number of choices increases even more. "Fixing" my physical health combines fixing my mental and spiritual health while trying to analyze how it all works inside. So, in a world of almost limitless choices, the questions *how do I know?* and *who do I listen to?* remain the most important ones.

Developing knowledge on many fronts while fostering a strong central core of self-care and self-practice works best for me. By now, you've surmised I'm not content trusting the advice of others. Trying solutions or combinations of solutions and seeing what works best has also worked well (as you'll see in chapter 21, When Bad Stuff Happens). The fact that I'm in this effort heart and soul with as little distraction as possible makes dealing with any health issues easier. My outside work takes second place to the core missions I have chosen as my priority.

THE ULTIMATE DIAGNOSTIC TOOL

Luckily, nature has given me the most exquisite diagnostic instrument ever created—my body with its sensory capacity. It includes my conscience—the place where head, heart, sense, and soul meet. With it, I can organize, prioritize, embrace, reject, analyze, and navigate the myriad amount of data and sensations I have at my fingertips about health. I can choose what works for me and what doesn't as well as evaluate others' advice to know what to incorporate into my practice and treatment. I don't blindly follow doctors' orders, knowing that they themselves disagree with each other. By studying the widest array of options, I can experiment with less invasive and more traditional treatments before deciding on any extreme measures.

"How *do* I feel?" My emotional biology is the starting place for everything. From there, I add knowledge gained from studies and reading, professional advice, and diagnostic results. I used to kid myself (or drink myself) into feeling "great" or "fine" when that wasn't true. Likewise, many times I would imagine the worst out of guilt or self-criticism. Now, the more I truthfully answer the question *how do I feel*—from my conscience and what I've learned—the more I have a grounded starting point from which to find solutions.

This is the essence of self-care—to make oneself the center of whatever practices, advice, and help is available in a quest to stay healthy and treat conditions that arise. As Eric Topol argues in *The Patient Will See You Now*, the basic relationship between patient and practitioner has started to radically change. This reality will be bolstered as preventive and integrative care practices become more accepted and commonplace. These practices already supplement doctors' traditional model of treating only symptoms and diseases; they're now *preventing* them as well.

DEFINING SELF-CARE

Before discussing diagnosis, treatments, and practices, let's look at the phrase "self-care"—care of oneself. *It means taking active responsibility for your health and your life.* It is being a benevolent parent or shepherd to yourself, a caring presence, a watchful guide. For me, how much I care for myself begins with how true I'm being to my inner voice, my inner spirit, my *ikigai*—the "sense of purpose" that has guided my journey since it began.

I hadn't actively cared about myself in that way for most of my life. Rather, my venture had been one of seeking approval of others, many times suppressing my own needs on their behalf. Today, the feeling of self-worth that ensues from caring for myself powers what I do to support myself—whether it's nutrition, movement, inner life, or other aspects of health noted in this book. These form a central core that's usually missing from a health program. And if any program is built on a foundation I don't believe in, then I know it will fall short of its goals. Actively caring for myself forms the heart of my whole mission.

CHANGE IN PERCEPTION OF DOCTORS

I have come a long way from my initial experiences with doctors (see chapter 3, Four Doctors). I now regard them as real, subjective people, not gods on high. I choose how I want to diagnose and treat myself during times of disagreement with them. This does *not* mean I don't go to doctors. Rather, I use them according to my own values without blindly following their advice as I once did.

I'm also passionate about avoiding drugs and surgery as much as possible, so I seek out doctors who respect this preference and will work with me on noninvasive measures. The more up-to-date doctors are, the more flexible they seem to be in this regard.

THE BASICS DEFINED

To recap, I've spent most of the past fifteen years achieving a baseline level of health I'm happy with. My definition of that baseline suits what I want from life and includes being as fully functional and healthy from a movement, flexibility, strength, energy, disease, psychological, and mental standpoint as I am able.

So far, it's working. At age seventy-three, most of my capacities are thriving better than before. I still watch out for and actively treat a right knee and hip problem and a heart arrhythmia. (Both these conditions and their treatment are discussed in chapter 21.) I regularly do strength and endurance tasks including seventy-three upside-down press-ups (yoga wheels or bridges) on my last birthday and a thirty-mile charity hike every year. I can no longer run fast or for any distance, but I never have been able to do that. Yet at the gym, I'm more flexible and can lift weights equal to many others half my age.

An example of my approach deals with my feet. Some time ago, I started having pain on the bottom of my feet. A podiatrist diagnosed a fallen arch and weak tendons—a condition called plantar fasciitis—and crafted custom arches to wear in my footwear. The arches quickly alleviated my pain, and I got used to wearing them. I noticed, however, that during the summer when I walked barefoot on grass, sand, and dirt, the condition disappeared. In fact, when I returned to wearing shoes and living in cities in the autumn, the condition didn't return for several months, but around midwinter, I had to go back to wearing the arches. I determined that my shoes and the hard pavements of cities had to be part of the problem.

So, I experimented with footwear that mimics walking as close to barefoot as possible. Known as "zero-drop" or "minimal" footwear, these shoes are equal height from the ground at the front and back. They're lightweight with adequate toe room to allow my feet to flex and grip while walking, thus simulating a barefoot experience. In addition, on long walks in parks and other outdoor places, I would walk on the ground or grass as much as possible, thus keeping engaged the intricate muscles in my feet and legs used for balance. The shoes also keep me more aware of the ground itself, our source of life.

This dramatic improvement was marked with only rare recurrences of the initial pain. I also increased my awareness of how my legs *feel* and I realized I've loosened the backs of my legs a great deal. (I can only imagine the extraordinary damage that high heels do, creating a highly exaggerated version of this problem.) I still wear the arches when the pain returns but can revert to living without them relatively quickly.

STARTING POINT AND DAILY METRICS

My day-to-day diagnostics begin with a morning routine. It starts with staying aware of what's going on in my body and my mind, not ignoring hints of possible problems, yet not exaggerating sensations that come and go. I'm not willing to write off my discomforts as "just getting old" or any other excuse. They need awareness or sorting out, especially if they persist. As Kelly Starrett writes in *Becoming a Supple Leopard*, "If it doesn't move, move it."

My finely tuned sense of inner dynamics has been enhanced more than ever. The power of concentration on specific body parts I've learned in yoga as well as other body sensations is central to this sense. "Breathing into a body part" is a tested yoga method to release tension. The well-being of all the parts in relation to each other is also central—a blessed awareness and powerful tool in the pursuit of health.

The heart rate variability (HRV) reading I take in the morning (see chapter 14) gives me a readiness score for activity that day, whether to actively train or recover. I don't trust it explicitly, for how I *feel* makes up part of the equation. Basically, I have a desirable high HRV for my age, averaging around 55–60 on this device, which indicates heart health as well as a favorable reading for longevity. (The average range for my age is lower—from 25–45.)

My morning breathing and movement routines provide opportunities for a diagnostic check-in. As I go through a range of movements along with deep breathing, an awareness of unusual stiffness or problems outside of yesterday's workout kicks in. I also check my mood and any lingering problems. Then I end the session with the Brazilian sitting exercise to assess balance, strength, and flexibility (see chapter 13) in which my score is 10 (or 9½ if I wobble a little). I want to do deep knee bends (even with a heavy weight) well into later life. To this end, I squat as far as I can so my butt almost touches the floor, and I hug my knees and get up several times. So far, so good.

ANSWERING HONESTLY

In addition to the physical realm, the questions *how am I doing?* and *how do I feel?* apply equally to my mental and spiritual state. It's always tempting to answer them positively, particularly in the company of others. However, the test is to answer them as honestly as possible, which might mean admitting that life isn't good at the moment and something needs to change. My emotional response to these questions directs this honest value system.

Admitting that life isn't as robust as it could be is *not* criticism. Rather, it's acknowledgement, acceptance, and movement from one stage to another. Fostering growth and moving through stuckness requires self-care, not self-hate.

LONG-TERM METRICS, RESEARCH, AND PROFESSIONAL HELP

Most metrics of my health result from being aware of how I am and what I can do almost daily. Having established that baseline level of health and making it a gift in my life helps me experience the joy of being alive. Nonetheless, other long-term metrics (some general and some specific to me) might show underlying or developing conditions. That's why I stay as current as possible on the latest studies and information, even though most don't surprise me.

As long as nothing specific is bothering me, I employ the variety of tests and procedures noted as follows.

Blood Tests

Once a year, I get a thorough complement of blood tests that includes vitamin and mineral panels as well as blood lipids and common regular medical testing. (See a full list of my regular tests in the Resources.) Some of the ultracelebrity health practitioners advise even more extensive tests than these. A purpose of these tests is to mark any changes in blood values and to gauge the balance of one level with others. Recognizing *how* and *why* any changes or imbalances become evident as well as whether results show a positive trend or not are important.

I do these blood tests independently with a lab or as part of a yearly check-up by my primary care physician. I keep test results for reference so I can decide which doctor needs to see them and for what purpose. To date, with one exception, I've never had surprises from any of them. The exception was a PLAC test for coronary plaque and the part of my heart journey I describe in chapter 21 in the section Fixing a Broken Heart.

Given my episode of heart arrhythmia, I also see a trusted cardiologist once a year and get an electrocardiogram, sometimes an ultrasound and stress test, plus a thorough coronary check-up. Every few years, I get a colonoscopy, as I have had several noncancerous polyps removed over the past fifteen years.

Research

In addition to these tests, I stay abreast of new areas of research, monitoring the state of the health and longevity community as well as reading about new studies, trials, and books. This includes some self-testing to see if new diagnostics or practices work for me. I keep weighing these against my current health practices and try them when they strike a chord.

Inevitably, I will encounter health problems that will affect my longevity. However, I believe paying maximum attention to *preventive* health one day at a time is the best way to take care of myself.

Support from Professionals and Others

When I'm as sincere, honest, and open as I can be with myself, I'm the only person who can know my issues well. My unconventional journey is one of radical self-care, shaped by the deepest part of me. The amount of self-knowledge that can come from my inner health journey invaluably helps with all areas of living, as I believe taking care of *health* is synonymous with taking care of *life*.

Doctors and other health professionals can be great assets when I don't succumb to the dependence and blind trust I once had. All doctors or health care providers come with their own subjective spin on issues. I want *my* subjective self-care to be part of that equation.

Having a qualified traditional MD is essential and the first step in turning to outside help. In my case, the MDs I work with must understand and support my mission as well as endorse the role of prevention and know why I'm pursuing it. They must respect my preference for staying off drugs and avoiding surgery; they take time for me; they discuss treatments candidly and understand when I say no to them. If something happens that requires intervention by modern medicine, I want *professionals who know me* to be on my side.

My specialty consultants also must conform to this model. When I turned to a specialist for my knee problem, for example, I was told that twenty years ago, doctors might have operated on my torn meniscus. Today, my specialist said patients do better with exercise, rehabilitation, and body strengthening rather than operations. I also work with an eye surgeon who gave me options before deciding about the best treatment. I *did* allow him to do surgery for a minor macular problem as well as a preemptive cataract-related lens replacement.

In addition, for anything invasive like the surgeon who did my heart surgery or the gastroenterologist I see for colonoscopies, I want to work with a great technician who communicates well. However, because I'm either asleep or numb while they do their jobs, I don't expect understanding and compassion. Rather, I demand what a professional airline pilot provides—someone thorough who has done this many times yet still pays attention to every detail, knowing that a life is at stake—*my* life.

Working with Nontraditional Providers

In addition to traditional doctors, I want to have nontraditional providers who become go-to resources on the prevention front. They keep up on the latest diet, supplement, and movement research as well as knowing what their own patients respond to.

In my case, I study everything from the *Harvard Medical School Health Guides* to the *Integrative Health Practitioners* news line to subscribing to prominent health and wellness practitioners and research services. (See Bibliography.) This information keeps me up to speed on new research. To build trust, I want my practitioners to know this research too, for I don't want to surprise them with details I've learned but they haven't.

Like traditional MDs, the nontraditional providers I work with are sympathetic to my views even if they don't always agree with me. In integrative health, I expect that the mind/body connection would be highly accepted by them. Because meditation has been shown to lower blood pressure as well as statins do, by 20 percent or more, an integrative practitioner should first know and then advocate using nonmedical means of treatment. Also, the best practitioners schedule long appointments, notice me as a person, and work to genuinely communicate with me and understand my preferences.

Therapy for My Inner Well-being

Therapy is in a special category (mentioned in chapter 15 on Clarity) that not everyone needs or wants (or can afford, given restrictions in healthcare), but it plays an important part in my life.

As described earlier, therapy requires paying attention to my inner life and staying open to inspiration and solutions. Lots of therapy is conducted (some at no cost) in the recovery movement through groups such as Alcoholics Anonymous (AA), Adult Children of Alcoholics (ACA), and related organizations. Often called "sharing," its purpose is to heal damaged inner lives.

For any treatment to be effective, though, it must be wanted. That requires an acknowledgment of suffering or simply stating that something needs fixing. It's also best practiced in harmony with self-effort and self-practice rather than treating it as a once-a-week exercise. *Being fully involved in healing is a 24/7 enterprise.*

The therapy process can be incredibly subtle, as it seeks roadblocks erected inside to keep me from seeing and feeling the truth. This is when a caring and knowledgeable therapist can provide expert support.

For much of my life, I was the president (and still a board member) of the board of the Karen Horney Clinic, a low-cost mental health clinic on New York's East Side. In this capacity, I have come to know many psychiatrists and psychologists. A skilled, trained practitioner can provide invaluable help navigating this terrain. That person could be a psychiatrist, psychologist, or counselor with whom a trusted relationship is built over time. As one of them told me, "Properly practiced, we end up holding souls in our hands."

Personally, I find commitment and trust essential to the success of the therapy process. It requires time, effort, patience, and honesty on the part of both of us. Without these essentials, therapy turns into paying someone to tell me I'm okay for an hour a week.

For me, the fruits of therapy have been invaluable. It has helped remove roadblocks inside I wasn't aware of and allowed growth, change, and feelings of vibrancy to flourish.

PART III

Fruits of the Journey

17

Parenting
A Universal Journey

"Theoretically, I can imagine that someday we will regard our children not as creatures to manipulate or to change, but rather as messengers from a world we once deeply knew, but which we have long since forgotten, who can reveal to us more about the true secrets of life, and also our own lives, than our parents were ever able to. We do not need to be told whether to be strict or permissive with our children. What we need to do is have respect for their needs, for their feelings, and their individuality, as well as for our own."
—ALICE MILLER

"And when I die and when I'm gone, there'll be one child born in this world to carry on."
—LAURA NYRO

As an older parent of young children, when I entered later life, I realized I'd be in a special category that few others find themselves in. Yet parenting is a universal journey, whether it's raising grandchildren, coming to terms with adult children, or being benevolent parents to ourselves and the eternal child within. Along with survival and reproduction, caring for our children is the most instinctual of our natural evolutionary drives. Perhaps it's even the most powerful; most parents would sacrifice their own lives for their children's.

Loving and nurturing my daughters continues to be the most rewarding experience of my life. Beyond just spending time and engaging with them, my connection with them is my biggest blessing ever. It's the spark that started my longevity journey as well as the inspiration to heal the trauma of losing and living without a father for most of my life. The self-worth that fuels my pursuit of health results from these dynamics.

But to be a better parent, I needed to explore my own childhood. Despite years of therapy, this was an inner journey I hadn't faced as deeply as I do today. I've come to realize how crucial and eternal the bond between parent and child is, in both healthy and unhealthy ways. It comes with an even greater responsibility for me to "get it right" with my own children in addition to being present, healthy, and connected.

Following are two stories that illustrate how I approached "getting it right."

PARENTAL PASS-ALONGS

This story involves my younger daughter, Lollie, who wanted to do something I had previously said she couldn't. I can't remember the details, which don't matter; the point is about saying no. She protested that it wasn't fair and started getting loud and angry. I reacted by becoming larger and louder myself to overpower her anger. I even shouted at her and threatened to make her go to her room if she didn't cool it. That raised her temperature even more. In response to her demanding, "Why? You're not being fair," I finally shouted in a near rage, "Because I'm the boss and that's what I said. Now go to your room until you cool off." I physically walked her there and closed the door, not too gently.

As soon as I did that, an image of my mother hitting me with a wooden spoon popped into my mind. She used to slam the door to my room and leave me alone to sulk. I recalled how unfairly treated, how un-listened to, and how weak I felt in the face of my mother's raging fits. She was forcing me to comply with her unexplained whims, making me feel afraid of her yet still dependent on her.

What was I most upset about with Lollie in this incident? Her protesting my orders, violating my power over her, and putting up her own courageous fight in the face of the injustice she felt. When I was her age, I feared my mother too much to protest. I would shrink and bend, forcing myself into submission rather than standing up to her.

All this took no more than fifteen seconds to sink in as these connections zoomed through me. *What am I doing? Why am I doing it? What damage have I done?* These questions couldn't begin to describe what went through my mind. I knew I had to change the conversation and repair what had just happened if I could.

So, I walked into Lollie's room and saw she'd buried her head in a pillow and clutched her favorite baby blanket for comfort. "Lol," I said, "I'm sorry. That was unnecessary, and you were treated unfairly. I'm sorry I got angry, and I just realized why I did that. That's what my mother used to do to me, and I felt awful when she did. But that's not an excuse, and I apologize to you. You didn't deserve that. Now let's talk." I had been rubbing her back as I said all this.

And we did talk. I explained why I didn't want her to do whatever she'd asked to do. We also worked out the timing of addressing other things first and then she could do what she wanted. I made the talk less arbitrary and dictatorial. Instead, I listened to her views and involved her in the decision-making process. Together, we made the issue feel fairer to her.

While this dynamic didn't disappear completely, future conversations and potential confrontations were less volatile after this one. More often than not, they were cut short and redirected by one of us once we realized we were headed into the same negative territory. They only very rarely, and briefly, happen now. The whole episode turned out positively for us both. It led me to realize how many of my parental actions I blindly pursued because of what had been done to me! Unwittingly, I was passing on that arbitrary unfairness and need for control to her. I realized that, until I became aware of my negative childhood experiences, I was powerless to change them.

THE BIRTHDAY GIFT

Another story involves Jessica, my elder daughter. I had given her a new bicycle for her tenth birthday. Because she looked forward to having the bike so much, we bought it in April (earlier than her actual birthday in June), so she could ride it and we could enjoy many lovely bike rides together before then.

Inspired by her riding, she planned a magnificent birthday party in the middle of London's Hyde Park. Her hand-picked spot bordered the small kiddie playground we used to go to; no doubt it triggered fond memories for her. Everyone invited—about ten of her favorite classmates and friends—would meet near Kensington Palace on their bikes or scooters. Then together, the group would ride through Hyde Park to the spot she'd picked. Waiting there would be a picnic my ex-wife had prepared, plus games and music and cake. Jess planned and created the whole day, partly inspired by a scene from an Angelina Ballerina book she liked.

PART III: Fruits of the Journey

On the morning of the big day, I woke up feeling tired and grumpy, having flown in from New York just a few days before. Although still jet lagged, I got up early to help with the party. As I made my way to the kitchen to prepare morning tea, I felt a resistance that was more than fatigue, and I admitted, "The last thing I feel like doing today is schlepping through Hyde Park with a bunch of ten-year-olds on bikes." This thought was followed by an almost immediate sensation in my gut. *What voice had just expressed those feelings?* Something inside needed to come to the surface. Feeling uncomfortable, I allowed it to percolate inside as I stared at the sky through our kitchen window.

What *were* these uncomfortable feelings? Then it dawned on me. *I was resenting my own daughter and the excitement of her day.* This wasn't aimed at her; it was *my* inner drama alone—and an insight that has shaped my parenting ever since.

My father died when I was seven years old and left a giant hole in my life. He had taught me how to ride a bike when I was five, much like I had done with Jess. Yet I never got a chance to enjoy the fruits of bike riding with him the way she would with me, especially on this day. The epiphany was that I noticed my resentment and anger of never having had his involvement in my childhood—feelings I'd been carrying around for decades but had nothing to do with my daughter. Had I not realized where they were coming from, they would have expressed themselves negatively during the day, at the very least as a bad mood. Once I allowed myself to feel my feelings and see the connection, my whole outlook changed. A deep emotional release followed. I remember thinking, *Wow! Jessica and her friends deserve the best day possible, and I can help make that happen.* Light and understanding remained where darkness and turbulence had been.

Even more, I realized I had deserved more of that kind of love and attention as a child. Along with renewed love for my daughter, I found compassion for my childhood self and what had happened to me. The fact that I hadn't received that kind of parental love made me no less deserving of it, then and now.

With newfound space, lightness, and buoyancy, I went to wake up Jessica on her special day. By overcoming the conflict of the previous minutes, I was able to provide my daughter with the opportunity I didn't have. My sluggishness disappeared, and I felt glowingly content to have helped this day happen for her.

In addition to marking a turning point in my parental understanding, this episode provided a springboard for seeing how invested I could be in suffering and resentment about what was missing in my childhood. This awareness gradually changed an old pattern into a new, freer one. I saw how this worked with others as well while it helped me experience more happiness and freedom than ever before.

TWO BIG LESSONS

Both these episodes taught me huge lessons. The first is that my childhood experiences and how I've continued to feel about them remain active players in my parenting. The emotions I experienced *then* are woven into the tapestry of how I experience life on many levels *now*.

I now know I have to pay attention to my childhood self in my relationships with my children. Their path to self-worth and freedom depends on my being aware of these subjective traps in myself. I either have to avoid them or air them out and deal with them. Freeing myself involves acting independently of my lingering buried life. I learned how quickly my mindset changes once I acknowledge what's going on inside, thus reinforcing how right it feels to do this work.

The second lesson has been to acknowledge that what I *don't* know about parenting far outweighs what I *do* know. I start by allowing my children to express themselves and be part of any conversation. Finding workable, cooperative solutions will be a never-ending challenge.

SELF-PARENTING REQUIRES CARING FOR MY INNER CHILD

By necessity, my personal work also involves being the best parent to *myself*. Were it not for this effort, the two episodes I described would have had different, less favorable outcomes. I realize that *how I relate to my children* and *how I relate to myself* are one and the same. Experiencing life genuinely and fully involves loving myself as well as loving them. In this regard, I've crafted my own version of the Golden Rule: *Do unto my children not only how I would do unto myself, but as I would have liked to be treated as a child.*

Self-parenting means engaging the loving, adult part of me to care for *my* inner child just as I provide the loving guidance I give my children. Both engage the same compassionate emotions and healing that allow me to feel new memories and experience physical renewal. I strive to let all these forces operate seamlessly and symbiotically within me.

NATURE TAKES OVER

Here I stand, the father of two teenage daughters who want and need to experience their lives on their own terms. What I've done to nurture that process serves as part of the foundation of their lives. But the vast work of becoming their own person is just beginning. I can keep watch over them, support them, and continue to coach and advise, yet ultimately, they take that giant step into the future on their own terms. What a wonderful journey for all of us, each in our own way!

I feel blessed to participate in their freshness and spontaneity. I delight in their imagination, direct play, and unconditioned interaction with the world around them. My goal? To let their spirits be as genuine as possible and not transfer my values onto them other than what they see by example and adopt for themselves.

Trying to rediscover the directness and freshness of childhood is the essence of Zen Buddhism and other spiritual practices. Later in life, many adults regret losing the spark they felt as children. My ultra-responsible, driven, hardworking, ambitious path began in my teens. While it brought me respect and a sense of importance, it also robbed me of the carefree experience of joy. Much of my time today is aimed at retrieving that joy. Allen Wheelis said it in his classic book *How People Change*:

> Adolescence, traditionally is the time of greatest freedom, the major choices thereafter being progressively made, settled, and buried, one after another, never to be reopened. These days, however, an exhumation of such issues in later life has become quite common, with a corresponding increase in freedom, which makes life again as hazardous as in youth.[1]

Many people I know regret their lack of ambition earlier in their lives and see the success that drove me as a good quality. Yet the compulsive, imbalanced quality I brought to those years became a rut in which I got stuck. Now in my later years, I strive to reclaim that lost freedom and creativity as well as the joy.

LOSING A CHILDHOOD

Recently, I talked with a palliative senior caregiver who looks after people in a special care home for nonfunctional seniors or terminally ill patients. He has a big heart for this challenging job. Many of the home's residents have dementia or Alzheimer's. Their bodies are still functional, but their minds are not.

In our conversation, he off-handedly said something profound—that most of these people focus their conversations not in the present but in the past. They talk to themselves or others about childhood memories as if their childhoods have taken over, leaving room for nothing else.

This deeply struck me. When a childhood gets lost, as part of mine did, something inside goes astray. Part of the soul gets lost, creating an imbalance. If that's not addressed and healed, that imbalance could stay locked up in the psyche and body, finding a way of expressing itself through dementia and other diseases. Perhaps among the contributors to increased disease in later life are unresolved, unhealed emotional scars from childhood. Perhaps lost children are crying to be heard. To the extent they didn't get what they needed in childhood, they have suffered and need to heal.

My journey continues to be the ultimate source for healing me and issues from my past. No doubt, my children will have their own issues to deal with as they mature. As a parent, a vital aspect of my job is appreciating life as part of a vibrant, healing universe and helping them see the path inside that's available for handling their issues—a path driven by self-value and self-love.

18

Modern Life
Friend or Foe?

> *"In primitive tribes, we observe that the old people are almost always the guardians of the mysteries and the laws, and it is in these that the cultural heritage of the tribe is expressed."*
> —CARL JUNG, *Modern Man in Search of a Soul*

> *"Simple pleasures are the best."*
> —BOBBY MCFERRIN

I was raised in the postwar baby boom when the promise of American life was unlimited in its ambition and scope. Yet it was all fueled by a relentless, and eventually rapacious, need for economic prosperity. This Mad Men panacea, which preyed on our subconscious desires for heaven on earth, appeared everywhere back then.

Until recently, I never learned the wisdom of what can come with having enough. I always needed more. I confused the *circumstances* of my life with the *quality* of my life. How others viewed me and my successes were deemed more important than my own gratification with those achievements.

THE BIG LIE OF NEEDING MORE

I have lived most of my life in the shadow of that dynamic—the big lie of needing more and doing more. Much of my journey has been evaluating my beliefs about what matters to me. I had been the poster boy for all the lavish "enjoyment" life offered—jetting back and forth to Europe, eating dinners in exclusive restaurants, drinking the finest wines money can buy. What's more, they became "necessary" in my role as the successful man with all the admiration that comes with it. The glow of activity close to the limelight and fueled by reinforcements like alcohol kept the dark side hidden from me. Having money became a prison in itself; most of my activities involved either new projects or different ways of spending it. I had to live up to these expectations, always upgrading aspects of my lifestyle—whether it was travel, a car or home or vacation house. "What's new, Ron?" always had an answer—a new project, a new purchase, or a new experience.

My social life revolved around the status of who I was *professionally* in business or in theater but not *personally*. Lots of those friendships faded, and only the real ones stayed solid once I sold the printing company and curtailed my theatrical work. I had probably passed on potentially valuable non-business friendships along the way. What happened?

My focus shifted entirely due to the experiences described throughout this book. I took off my mask. I no longer went from one project to another; I no longer put effort into maintaining my public and social self. With no mask, I realized I had been terrified of finding the real person underneath and had used my careers as a crutch. Yes, I still employ my abilities and talents and creativity in pursuit of what I want. I have, however, changed the focus.

Conventions of modern life—everything from misinformation to fear of being different and my attachment to them—still form much of the resistance in the work I do today. I've found that all the past affluence and achievements don't come close to the inner peace and joy of one day of simple pleasure and robust health I have now—of being a father to my children, working on my current practice, and just appreciating being alive.

WHAT COULD BE

Don't get me wrong; I acknowledge and am grateful for the safety and convenience of modern life. Without worrying about my next meal and having a secure roof over my head, I could not have the time and/or leisure to take this journey of longevity. I've had to *re*-discover and *re*-learn the world of health, knowing that *nothing about acquiring more stuff will help me on this path*.

In many ways, modern life itself never needed fixing; it's my *buying into it* that had to change. Time and again, I come back to my natural, ancestral, evolutionary, and universal ways. Fostering my health and its origin integrates all the key elements and gives me a basis for what works and what doesn't. I used to take in much of the modern messaging without question. Once I looked under the hood—at those messages as well as myself—I realized the vastness of the unquestioned health beliefs within me.

FOCUS ON PREVENTION

I've noticed many articles, programs, and documentaries showing natural remedies like diet and exercise are as effective (if not more so) than medical treatment for health problems. Any shift toward preventive medicine takes time and involves inner change. However, no amount of advice or reasoning can get someone to make this shift. It needs to start *inside*. People must *want* to change so they can be in better health—or get scared by a health emergency that *forces* them to want better health.

As this trend continues, functional medicine and integrative healthcare, which advocate noninvasive, preventive treatment as alternatives to traditional medical solutions based on drugs and/or surgery, become more popular. Qualified practitioners, many of them MDs, have become frustrated with Western medicine's adherence to drug and surgical treatments. Even those at the forefront of traditional medicine realize that the power to heal lies within us and needs to be activated through better health habits.

For example, a *Scientific American* article[1] by Avery Posey, Carl June, and Bruce Levine titled "A New Model for Defeating Cancer: CAR T Cells" noted the biggest breakthroughs in cancer research and treatment have come in the field of T cells. They activate the body's own immune system to fight the cancer. Instead of invasively aiming to destroy cancer cells with chemotherapy or radiation, getting our own bodies to fight the disease is at the forefront of most research.

My practice represents a daily experiment in *what works for me*. Comparing it with other people's ways of improving their health, these preventive measures have much in common. They are based on adopting a simpler, more conscious lifestyle with more movement and a more natural, less manufactured diet than before. And many people are realizing their beliefs and inner lives are integral to their overall health. Whether therapeutic or preventive, these tenets become starting points.

Modern medical professionals and the medical-industrial complex fight this view. Their message is "go ahead and live an unhealthy life and we will fix you." As a result, one's life can become a vicious cycle that relies on conveniences such as drugs, surgery, and endless stuff to buy. They keep the illusion alive that *progress is always good for us*. Yet, by living simpler, more natural lives, eating natural foods, and moving more, many of these treatments and remedies wouldn't be necessary in the first place. It begs this question: *How much of modern medicine treats conditions being caused by living the way we do?*

FOOD INDUSTRY'S CONTROL OVER FOODS

At an Integrative Healthcare conference in New York, I heard Dr. Mark Hyman, head of the Ultra Wellness Center and noted author, outline the extreme control that the US food industry holds over the quality and choice of foods available. This is a topic he explores further in his book *Food Fix*. Not only do a handful of companies own all the so-called "healthy" brands; they constantly wage battles to obfuscate information and lobby governments and organizations to use their products despite increasing evidence that *overusing* them is a primary cause of illness. Sugary drinks, for example, are still being served in many schools based on monetary contributions drink companies make to organizations that run the schools. Like the practices for which the tobacco industry was finally held accountable, doing this is downright dishonest.

As food author Michael Pollan advised, the solution needs to be consumer driven—something that leads to *better individual awareness and practice*. What are good practices? To eat food that doesn't come in a box or was made in a factory or is a suspicious-looking "food" product. "Something your great grandmother would recognize as food," he writes. I suggest learning what is a healthy diet and what is not, then changing your buying behavior, which can be the best way to change the industry's behavior. Corporations will be forced to change if consumers stop purchasing their products.

Still, I know it's a big battle to fight. The behavioral tentacles that come with advertising, the monolithic control of these companies, and the societal and parental pressure we're exposed to from an early age make this change more difficult than ever.

EVOLUTIONARY MISMATCH AND THE WORLD UNTIL YESTERDAY

Riddles are less puzzling when they're studied from the perspective of humanity's evolutionary past. Even in our "prehuman" past, writers such as Mary Midgley in *Beast and Man* eloquently show the seamlessness and gradualness with which evolutionary "leaps" have occurred. We live today with many ancient evolutionary systems and emotional architecture still in place. Our inability, and at times refusal, to acknowledge we even have this prehistoric history make these realities hard to grasp. We have a hard enough time reimagining civilizations two thousand years ago that have been passed down in written form—let alone two million or so years ago when we began walking on two legs.

Two of my favorite places to study our prehistoric past are books by Daniel Lieberman and Jared Diamond. I have summarized their concepts here.

The term "evolutionary mismatch" comes from Daniel Lieberman's *The Story of the Human Body*. In it, he details the evolutionary march our bodies have taken to get where we are now. Almost all this journey has been under nature's dominion, directed by the sacred program called evolution. Hopefully, humans will spend just as many eons trying to unravel, respect, and be grateful for this process. Only in the past infinitesimally short period—the equivalent of less than a tenth of a second in a twenty-four-hour day—have we been living anywhere close to the modern lives we do today.

The result of this vast technological, cultural, and environmental transformation has been to change how our bodies have thrived for all our existence. This radical change in such a short period is the underlying cause of much of what we call illness. Yet somehow, we largely believe we were made for *this* world and not *that* one. Evolution cannot work at that speed. Activity, or lack thereof, that's out of sync and balance with why our bodies were originally made form the core of his arguments.

Here are Lieberman's four basic symptoms of these mismatches:

1. **Disease**. As was documented in modern hunter-gatherer studies, illnesses like cancer and heart disease were rare to nonexistent. On the other hand, infections and accidents caused injury and death. Some people believe humans have more disease because we live longer. Lieberman showed that this argument doesn't hold up; rather, much of today's lifestyle fosters our modern symptoms and diseases.
2. **Too much**. Too much energy force-fed into bodies that evolved on hunger and leanness causes a great amount of disease today. Our bodies were made to store as much nutrition as possible in the form of fat, a trait that helps us survive when availability of food is scarce. Humans were not made to dwell in the "land of milk and honey" in which food is available 24/7, with regular mealtimes, almost constant consumption, and easily absorbed and excessive sugar- and starch-based diets. If that fat we store never gets used, it ends up as permanent fat, which clogs and slows down an otherwise highly dynamic system. Hunger also provided the prod to find food, to move. Hunger also caused us to become stronger, better, and more inventive at what

we did, which primarily was looking for food. Modern life encourages our appetite for many things to become insatiable and for us to eat all the time without the effort involved in securing our food. This is not our evolutionary heritage.

3. **Disuse.** We used to move more and walk up to ten miles a day while also doing strenuous hunting, foraging, and later farming. We sat on the ground, got up and down all the time, and used our bodies for everything. We are now even hard pressed to carry our groceries home.

4. **Novelty and comfort.** Lieberman found convincing problems with everything from comfortable shoes to eyeglasses to chairs to soft foods that don't need chewing to digest. Our pursuit of comfort and novelty further distances our bodies from being used the way they were meant to. This generates more disuse and misuse of the vital systems that keep us alive.

DAMAGE OF MODERN LIFE ON A PSYCHIC AND CULTURAL LEVEL

Although beyond the scope of his book, Lieberman omits the damage that modern lifestyles cause on a psychic and cultural level. However, Jared Diamond addresses some of this in *The World Until Yesterday*. On the same evolutionary timeline, Diamond explores the social norms of our ancestors and contrasts them with today's evolved systems. He does this through his vast experience in Papua, New Guinea. In just a few generations, people there have undergone a transformation that has taken the Western world thousands of years. Diamond was one of the first anthropologists to discover some of the first Neolithic tribes in their initial encounters with the outside world. Many of them still live this way, although the changes that the outside world have brought them have been seismic.

Reading his book, I was struck by several themes—especially the norms these people established in their own natural, organic way without the help of contemporary laws, economies, or institutions. They put in place highly effective and moral practices to deal with all sorts of tribal governance specific to their lifestyle and belief systems. These tribes hold great lessons for us today. Discarding them as "primitive" and thinking our ways are better would be a big mistake.

Here are two of their most poignant practices:

1. **Justice.** This is a system to deal with crime that has survived from tribal days into the present. The case example Diamond used was a boy's accidental death caused by a driver from a different clan. Afterward, both families and clans, led by the elders of each clan, worked together to find a fair solution. They arrived at one after hearing everyone out and allowing them to vent their emotions and views. The solution involved a ceremony to pay respect to the dead boy, and members of both clans attended it. The aim was to keep peace and avoid revenge that could have resulted in violence. They also came up with a fair compensatory settlement and an apology to the boy's family. All this was accomplished by the ceremony, an admission, apology, and compensation from the driver as well as public forgiveness from the boy's family. The civil authorities only got involved after this settlement was reached. They charged the man with reckless driving, fined him, and suspended his license. Diamond contrasts this approach with the vengeful,

punishment-oriented, impersonal, and defensive sense of court justice commonly practiced today.

2. **Treatment of the young and the old.** Once they can walk, children in these and other indigenous tribes are more autonomous than those in our society would tolerate. In particular, they're allowed to play with knives, fire, and other dangerous objects. Learning by injury and surviving is the time-tested way they are taught.

On the other hand, they are closer than us to their mothers and other tribe members in their first two years until they learn to walk. Constantly in contact, infants are exclusively breastfed until they want other food or can learn to find it themselves. On this note, I was once struck by a documentary about a Brazilian tribe in which children around five years old went into the forest alone. At that age, they already knew to avoid certain poisonous spiders and snakes, and they happily snacked on bugs, caterpillars, and tasty leaves along the way.

In these tribal societies, the elderly are treated much differently than in our modern society. The elderly are looked up to, admired for their wisdom, and usually act as the arbiters of disputes. Their wisdom is especially venerated. They're expected to carry their load and keep up with others—no special treatment—until they can't. They are also expected to transmit their wisdom to younger clan members. When they can't do that anymore, they are left alone to die or live by themselves until they do pass. For them, death is an acknowledged part of life.

Diamond's look at this "prehistoric" world has fascinated me. It is far from a wholesale rejection of modern life, yet it gives us pause to consider the advantages of taking elements from both the modern and traditional worlds.

Much can be said in favor of today's evidence-based approach that has brought us advances in science and knowledge. Yet the world I was exposed to when I allowed myself to be guided by *inspiration* as well as *reason* has become my life now. And it is far richer and more wholehearted than how I lived before. Much of modern life asks us to discard, or at least ignore, a lot because emotions are not as neat as facts and figures. Yet people can suffer greatly in this regard, so by allowing ourselves to awaken inside provides a primary path to better health in all respects. And this brings me again to the main subject of this book—*genuine inner change*. How do I change in ways that align with my genuine inner self and that go beyond mere willpower?

THE ROAD LESS TRAVELED

I know of no other way to improve my health and fix my misguided reliance on aspects of modern living than to follow the signposts of my newly awakened internal life. This has proven to be a reliable, albeit challenging, path through the thickets of my inner experiences. My appreciation of its power began on that train ride to New Jersey, a moment of deep inspiration coming from nowhere yet reaffirmed time and again as a true path for me.

But this path is hardly conventional. For a long time, I felt like an outcast on a lonely journey. The growing strength I was being granted kept me going. Now, after many years, I have been able to put my experiences into conversations in a way that's appreciated by others.

I have found that loneliness, feeling different than other people, and needing to alleviate those feelings are my three biggest obstacles to adopting an attitude of self-benevolence. For me, feelings of anxiety or discomfort are regular features of life. When this happens, I know there is a self-critical dynamic at work inside me, and I encourage myself to endure the anxiety and feel all my feelings as deeply and genuinely as possible. I know they are vestiges of the emotional trauma I experienced in my childhood. At the same time, I pray and ask for a way through the darkness, some sort of resolution. This practice almost always leads me to higher ground and more light if I allow it the time and power it needs.

Once clarity comes, it not only allows me more freedom and inner space, it also sheds light on the original experience that triggered the self-criticism. My roots in this soil lie deep in the world of being an only child combined with the trauma of losing my father at an early age. Yet, I have taken great comfort in what I've read or witnessed in people I admire, past and present. I've learned that the arduous work of inner change and self-discovery is almost always a solitary pursuit. Joseph Campbell documents similar journeys through the world of religion and mythology. Richard Bucke tells of a kind of universal spiritual awakening in many historical figures from Buddha to Walt Whitman in his book *Cosmic Consciousness*.

Defying conventional ways leads to self-integrity and self-discovery. Not accidentally, this path has also best served my health and longevity pursuits. It has given me an internal anchor to ground my journey through the advice minefields out there.

MY SELF-REALIZATION

My journey is about finding the unique wonder of my own self, appreciating where I came from while nourishing the source through which I experience the world. My existence depends on a web of interconnected systems, inside and outside, natural and societal, that support me. Without them, I couldn't live.

Modern life let the genie of self-conscious individuality out of the bottle. My individuality was made possible by eons of tribal life—human beings welded together looking out for the tribe's survival using their collective humanity. Any personal need was submerged to the tribe's need—as often prevails in clan cultures as well as families. Individuality could only emerge once basic needs of food and shelter became relatively assured and were universally accessible.

As a species, we are still coming to grips with this new power of consciousness. We aim to integrate it into the preexisting history of being told how to act by our DNA. For the first time in the span of the cosmos we are able to choose how to act differently. Much of this new power has gone to our heads. We believe we can master our lives apart from the natural world. To this extent, we have distanced ourselves from nature in many ways such as believing food comes from a supermarket instead of the soil and the earth.

A parallel process also takes place inside us. To the extent we rely on reason and logic and ignore or override our emotions, we are denying the nature inside us. This is complex and subtle work.

Self-realization is about experiencing this terrain, the 90 percent of each of us that is below the surface. Changes in that realm have shifted the way I experience the world around me. That subjectivity is the dark, secretive treasure of self-realization. It is light, the inner promised land addressed by many religions. Ultimately, *it happens when our inner life is integrated in a balanced way with thought, feeling, and spirit harmonizing with the world around us.* Self-realization is not a steady state of bliss as I once imagined nirvana to be; it's a dynamic and ever-changing landscape that swells and crashes as much as it brings us peace and calmness. The ultimate source of health and inspiration, it lives and breathes. It's alive with possibility, and it's endlessly evolving.

A PILOT'S STORY

I have a friend who has spent his life as an airline pilot. He loved what he did and misses it terribly. He was forced to retire due to a mandatory corporate retirement age, despite still performing to the same level on the high-intensity simulator exercises pilots are given. He was also robbed of his pension by a corporate bankruptcy. During his career, he safely piloted over four hundred thousand passengers and flew over ten million miles. Just think of how we take professionals like him for granted when we fly—yet we trust our lives to them every time.

A lifetime of having to sit in a cockpit for a living has left my friend with a stiff back and limited mobility, none of which he ever foresaw, budgeted for, or attempted to treat preventively with his employer and healthcare. His regular doctor said he was "just getting old" at sixty and prescribed painkillers and anti-inflammatories, which he decided to put off. His preferred solution has called for rebuilding his life at this age. He began to meditate, went to beginner yoga classes, and started sharing his feelings more openly.

Like many others, he had put his faith in our modern world and now sees the downside of having lived that way. He has a deep current of feeling discarded and resentful. Yet short of "fixing" our society, his only path to joy—like all of ours—is to fix what's not working for him.

19

Vanity

Attempts to Look Young

"We are all meant to shine as children do."
—MARIANNE WILLIAMSON

Like the temptations of modern life, vanity has exerted a tug on my resources for years. If there ever were a time to *not* be vain, it's in later life when the race to look other than I do becomes impossible. As I'm with others my age, those who impress me most are the people who have an inner life and/or a healthy and fit body—something I can see in their eyes, their faces, their posture, and their movement. They "shine," as Marianne Williamson says in the quote above.

TIME TO SHINE

Yet old habits die hard. The reinforcements that surround us are always present, including actors and models being advice givers and spokespeople for products claiming they will make us look younger. They still sometimes get the better of me when I confuse *appearance* with being *valuable and loveable*. Even at seventy-three, I feel proud when people tell me I look much younger than my age. But this has nothing to do with beauty treatments or adjusting my appearance.

It has everything to do with tending to my life inside, where health begins. What appears on the *outside* reflects the healthiness *inside*.

Nature built us to pair, bond, and reproduce. We select a mate based on many subtle factors, appearance being one of them. This is normal. Sexual and loving attractions are astronomically complex, age-old riddles we won't figure out or rise above anytime soon. We can only answer the puzzle inside ourselves. The myth of Narcissus is 2,500 years old and remains as fresh as ever.

Looking back, the best, most genuine, long-lasting compliment I've received about my appearance happened in my early thirties after I started selling printing. A client whom I hadn't seen in a few months remarked, "Whatever you've been doing on the inside, it shows on the outside. You look great." I had indeed been struggling yet had begun to realize my strengths in a business I cared about. I passionately wanted to succeed and had worked hard to do so. Around that time, I had started therapy and began work on my "underground dynamics," notably my self-criticism. He perceptively saw the change in my demeanor and how it affected my appearance. He became my biggest client for a time, and we became good friends as well.

ONE DAY AT A FLORIDA GYM

When I was sixty-four, I went to visit my then eighty-year-old aunt who lives in a Century Village complex in Florida. One day I used the gym there and then went to a large, empty studio to stretch and do yoga. At one point, I lay down on the floor, and what did I see? Taped to the studio ceiling were beefcake magazine pinups of hot, muscled men. I could only imagine what they were doing there. Indeed, a trainer I saw on the way out confirmed that the photos help motivate some of the women to try harder. The message was clear: "C'mon, ladies, don't you want to have a body that someone like that wants to be with?"

I laughed and scratched my head. Yet the gym I go to is full of young men and women who believe the same thing when they "body sculpt" and "pump iron." Mirrors are everywhere. They want to look better to attract or keep love in their lives—an age-old desire that won't change anytime soon.

A traditional alternative to this was reflected in an interview I saw with a woman in the Hadza, a hunter-gatherer tribe in Tanzania. When asked about her ideal man—wasn't he one of the young, good-looking men of the tribe?—she laughed. Her ideal man, she said, was older, wiser, and a good hunter who was able to provide. Looks had nothing to do with it!

OBSESSED WITH IMAGE

We live in an era obsessed with image. In this society, we confuse our appearance with our ability to be loved, and we even tragically blame how we look when we are *not* loved. Questions like "what's wrong with me?" or "why can't I look like that" start in our teens or earlier and usually never leave. Looks become a notch on the "I'm not good enough" belt as we assume models or celebrities lead much "better" lives than us.

In my theatrical career, I've known celebrities whose public lives are depicted in the media as glamorous and charmed. I know first-hand that, despite their talents, they are all normal human beings in private, with as messy and conflicted inner lives as anyone else. Yet the cult of celebrity and envy prevails today more than ever.

Accepting who I am and how I look, genuine and unjudged, is what I strive for. When it comes to appearance, my mantra is *to work on the inside* and, as far as the outside goes, "It is what it is."

Attempts to Look Young

Put aside the fact that remedies for wrinkles and other old-age eventualities treated by cosmetics, surgery, and fashion don't work. Several dermatologists and even a cosmetics executive I spoke to in confidence have told me this: "We're selling dreams." Their tools are words and scents and textures and procedures. But the amount of time pursuing false beauty ideals as the basis for love robs us of precious time to do the things that actually work—movement, diet, reflection, and cultivating our inner spirit. On a macro scale, the amount of money and time spent on these ineffective treatments is simply wasted.

Older people can experience this vanity doubly hard. We get dismissed as weak, not desirable, not sharp, not needed, and not up to date. But the place to fight this ageism is inside ourselves, not outside. To the extent I allow myself to be taken in by the attitudes of others, I become a victim of them. The roots of my feelings go all the way back to childhood, especially my teenage years when being attractive seemed to define everything about popularity. I've spent decades in the throes of insecurity about my appearance, dating models and actresses to complement my successful lifestyle. Only now am I finding relief in a genuine inner experience. My appearance no longer matters.

The Real Me

So, who am I? Over the past fifteen years, the answer to that question is as profoundly endless as any other mystery in the universe. *I am more than I thought I was when I began.* Most important, I am more than who I see in the mirror and any image I once had of myself. When I think of vanity and mirrors, I'm reminded of that classic *New Yorker* cartoon of the matronly woman who only sees her young, beautiful reflection in the mirror. That reflection resides in her psyche, her own highly subjective and inaccurate version of what she wants to look like as the perfect vision of beauty and youth.

To the extent there is a "real me," it's no longer the accomplished image I have of myself striding through the world, nor is it the devastated little boy who lost his father and whose life turned upside down at that moment. Despite their lasting presence and influence on my life today, these images are part of me, but *I am not them.*

Rather, I've become a more genuine version of myself. I no longer need to please others to have them love or admire me. I no longer need to be successful in their eyes but only as it matters to me. I am a living, breathing, visceral soul whose self-worth and validity were provided at birth. Yes, my self-worth did get knocked down, but I am reclaiming it in my later years.

How others will remember me pales compared to my new life inside, my "here and now" experience with its awe, wonder, aliveness, curiosity, and health. I regard my physical appearance as a product of my inner life, not the other way around.

20

Genes
The Role They Play

"Genes and family may determine the foundation of the house, but time and place determine its form."
—JEROME KAGAN

We are lucky to be living in an age of increasingly vast knowledge about our genes. Although research is still in its infancy, we know specific genes might predispose us to certain diseases, rather than simply guessing based on our family history. More important, we know that having potentially harmful genes is not a sentence that can't be changed by lifestyle and belief. The field of interaction between our conscious choices and nature's programs holds great promise, not only for our health but for evolution in general. We know that genes and DNA coding, the basis of evolution, can be changed—although to what extent remains to be explored.

At the center of this work lies the conditions that turn our gene expression mechanisms on and off. Having a potentially harmful genetic trait does not necessarily mean it plays an active role, which is similarly true with favorable traits that don't get turned on. Lifestyle, movement, and diet have some effect. But fascinating to me is *epigenetics*, the way our activities affect the genes inherited by our offspring. *This is the core of how evolution transmits favorable traits to generations that follow.*

Inevitably, moral and political dilemmas such as *how* and *how much* genes could or should be altered will spark debates for decades. But for my focus on health and longevity, I'm encouraged by what I have discovered, both personally and in my practice and research.

MY GENETIC STORY

My own genetic story differs from that of most people. Because I was adopted at birth, I knew nothing about my genetics for most of my life. By digging and doing a genetic test, I found out a few things, yet I had many unanswered questions.

I'm glad I don't have the genes of my adoptive parents, both of whom died young of cancer—my father at age forty-seven from pancreatic cancer and my mother a few weeks shy of her fifty-sixth birthday from ovarian cancer. In some respects, being adopted has allowed me to approach my health and longevity goals in a more clinical, independent way.

SEARCH FOR MY BIRTH MOTHER

Over time, I've found information about my genetics and my birth parents, most of which is encouraging. From papers I found after my adopting mother died, I learned my birth mother's maiden name and where I was born—Montreal, Canada. I also learned that *she* had given me my first and middle names, not my adopting parents.

My prearranged adoption happened immediately at birth, although my mother never told me that when she shared the standard story of my being "chosen." For a long time, I never felt a need to pursue the matter. Then, about twenty-five years ago, through a serendipitous coincidence, I found not only my birth mother's new married last name and address but her age and health history as well. Her health history showed no serious illnesses, which was good news for me. One surprise, though, was learning she gave birth to me in her midthirties; she wasn't the much younger woman I had imagined. My girlfriend at the time persuaded me to write her a letter saying my life was turning out fine. "There is not a day that goes by that she doesn't think of you," my girlfriend assumed. "Knowing your life has been good will be good news to her, especially as she gets older." So, I sent the letter but never heard back from her.

Although some people advised me to pursue this and others said not to, in the end I didn't. Finding out her health history was a bonus, and I left it at that.

"23 AND ME" TEST

My interest stayed dormant for a long time, but as my health and longevity practice grew, I became more curious about my real genetics. So, I took a "23 and Me" test a few years ago. This is a DNA test showing genes that might predispose me to disease and what my evolutionary heritage is made up of (i.e., where my ancestors came from). The results indicated I had no genetic predispositions or elevated risks for any diseases. A subsequent, more specific test using data for my genetic sports profile showed I was intolerant of carbohydrates, that I fared better with a high-fat, low-carbohydrate diet, and that my aerobic profile was extremely favorable. That meant I was naturally inclined to move a lot. Although I'd lived with this information on a sensory level all my life, my genes now reinforced it!

I decided that finding out more about my genetic history might be useful to my daughters in addition to getting their own testing done. My mission got bigger!

I found a listing for my birth mother in the Montreal White Pages and wrote another letter. This time, I said I needed information for my children, especially about my biological father. Could she help? Again, I got no response, although I know this letter and a follow-up one were both delivered and signed for as registered mail. At this point, she was in her late nineties, so even if she wasn't capable herself, whoever opened her mail could have replied.

Still curious, I picked up the phone and called. Amazingly, she answered. At first, I asked her if that was her maiden name. "Yes," she replied. Then I told her my name, and she immediately recognized it. "Oh, are you in town?" she asked. I told her I wasn't in Montreal but that I had sent her letters about who I was and why I was calling. She seemed confused and said very abruptly, "I know exactly who you are, and I'm not interested." Then she hung up.

That was our last contact. I decided not to pursue it. Yet a few years later I searched the internet and saw her obituary in a Montreal paper. She had died of natural causes at age 103. As much as failing to reunite with her caused me pain, the silver lining was knowing about her longevity—which bodes well for me, my daughters, and my mission.

GENES AND LONGEVITY

The subject of genes and longevity always gets raised when the Blue Zones and other longevity hotspots are discussed. I believe there's more to longevity than genes and nature, though. Lifestyle in the form of movement, diet, attitude, belief, outlook, and purpose all play equally large roles. Then there's nurturing, even in the form of witnessing your parents staying active into their eighties and nineties.

Still, genes play a part that can't be discounted, even though the hard predeterminism some people give them is probably overstated. The more that healthy lifestyles are practiced and documented, the less credence science gives to genetic factors. If we lived in a world of mass health consciousness and active health practice, especially in later life, scientists would do proper studies on longevity and genetics, and we'd learn more about how *nurture* influences *nature* in humans.

MY GENETIC FATHER

For some reason, I never felt the need to search for my genetic father. Maybe it was because I had no real place to start but also because I felt more loved by my adopting father (despite his short life span) than I ever did by my adopting mother. And maybe my search for an alternative father was not as important as finding another mother.

Then one day, I got a serendipitous message from the universe that opened a new door. I received a notice from "23 and Me" about my DNA relatives. Notices usually point to third or fourth cousins, which could include many, many people. But one person showed up as a first cousin who had a 7 percent DNA match with me. This high percentage indicated a close genetic relation—that is, we have a grandfather in common. So, I requested having her contact me to share information.

Unlike the maternal side of my genetic family, she wrote back in an extremely open, sympathetic, and helpful way. I quickly learned that, when it comes to birth heritage, DNA doesn't lie. After I sent her a picture of me, she replied, "Oh yeah, you're one of us. I can see it in your face and everything about you. Welcome to the family!"

We worked through various possibilities stemming from this large extended family. It was full of siblings and half siblings due to our common grandfather remarrying after his first wife died prematurely. (It turns out I was her half first cousin.) In the end, we determined which of the grandfather's sons was my father.

I have now corresponded with all my new stepsiblings, and we've shared details about our lives. They told me that our father, who had died about ten years before of complications from diabetes, was a loving, caring, curious, and independent soul. He loved music and children; he was always making new friends with quirky but fascinating people. He didn't suffer fools or bullshit. And we still haven't figured out how he and my birth mother got together before either of them married—probably a mystery forever. Although I haven't met these stepsiblings face-to-face, getting to know them has been a satisfying chapter in my life.

SCARS OF ADOPTION

Some psychologists argue that the scars of adoption—of never being able to attach to the physical birth mother you were part of for nine months—last a lifetime. That view applies even to early adoptions like mine because the subconscious mind is powerful enough to retain that emotional memory. My truth is that I didn't get the love I needed from either my birth mother or my adoptive mother. Therefore, my genetic journey is one of parenting as well as DNA and about how the lasting effects of adoption change children's lives. This brings the lessons of my journey squarely back to my daughters and my own mission to heal and stay healthy for them.

Since life began, DNA and genes have been at the center of evolution, forming the pathways by which everything gets transmitted to the next generation. Classic Darwinian evolution holds that "random" mutations in genes—slight changes in the complex chemical makeup of these tiny strands of protein—are responsible for evolutionary changes.

I don't agree. It's hard to believe anything so precious to life in our ever-evolving universe is random. I come back to the notion of *a sacred direction* to evolution, a mysterious, complex, and subtle dance of "ever-improving" (another phrase for healing) that the universe has been doing forever. The latest iteration of that improvement is us humans. Our consciousness has been given to us to figure out how to continue surviving. We can't know this evolutionary plan in advance; all we can do is live it, appreciate it, and harmonize with it.

I believe a direct line of connection exists between the actions of a person and the DNA passed into offspring. It's like evolution is one big trial-and-error machine, with the best solutions making changes to improve the next generation. The lives we lead, our actions, and our beliefs are the source of those DNA "mutations." Better survival for our species and the chance to continually evolve is the *only* bottom line the universe understands. If the changes improve the next generation's chance of survival, they'll stick. If not, they'll succumb and die off.

My very existence has been made possible by the eons of infinite DNA changes since the first life took form on our planet. And my genes contain the record of all the evolution that has taken place since then.

NOT SUCCUMBING TO FEAR

If my version of the universal power of healing is remotely true, then freedom is everything DNA is about—specifically the freedom to change, improve, and serve the organism it's part of. Its opposite—fear—fuels any belief that we can't escape our genetic destiny.

Of course, we will all die one day. Yet living with the flame of life burning brightly until then is what I am after. The effort, belief, and faith I have discovered on my path are my ultimate allies in *not* succumbing to fear. This doesn't mean never feeling afraid; it simply means there is something *alive and wonderful* on the other side of fear.

Since that fateful train ride, I continue to find my way through that sometimes-dark forest. It's what real life is all about for me now.

21

When Bad Stuff Happens
Three Lessons in Healing

"Old age ain't no place for sissies!"
—BETTE DAVIS

This chapter features three lessons I've learned about health from three serious conditions, any one of which could have derailed my quest for longevity and vitality. I engaged with each condition on every level I could to find solutions. My body and my being helped me (somewhat miraculously) figure out how to heal and/or stabilize them as well as who to seek for expert advice. The extraordinary degree of integration within me steered the process of tapping as many resources as I could. The conditions I share affecting my right leg and hip, my heart, and my whole body via an acute case of Lyme disease have all healed or stabilized, but they made me aware of vulnerabilities that needed attention. And I was able to restore my full health without resorting to ongoing medication or medical treatment.

LESSON ONE: LEARNING TO WALK AGAIN

About five years ago, I started feeling soreness and pain in my right hip and knee. It didn't lessen with any of my regular practices. Over a few weeks, the pain affected my ability to walk. I might easily have chalked it up to old age as I've seen others do and sought a traditional medical fix. But then, my entire later-life journey might have crashed and burned. Instead, after having the situation thoroughly checked out medically, I've discovered remedial, nonmedical solutions that have returned full use to those parts of my body, albeit with occasional discomfort. Had I not put in the effort and done the research earlier, the nonsurgical and nonpharmaceutical alternatives would not have been in my health toolbox.

These solutions also addressed other areas of my hips, spine, and body that I had no idea were affected. Imbalances I was compensating for had already started developing in my posture. The integrated organism that is me was compensating for the reduced strength in my leg. On the way to restoration, other hidden mental and emotional components became evident.

In addition to my knee and hip, the front of my right thigh was sore. After some online "Dr. Google" research, I came up with a common complaint among runners called "IT syndrome," which seemed to fit the bill. "IT" is short for *iliotibial band*, a sheath of tendon wrapped in fascia running from the outer hip to the outer knee. It can become inflamed with overuse or injury. That happens when an area bears an extra load due to weak glute and hamstring muscles and associated tendons in the hips, buttocks, and legs.

I had been running at that time, an activity I wasn't used to and have never been good at. Specifically, I was doing wind sprints as one of my high-intensity rotations, running as hard as I could for about 100 yards and then walking back. This took great effort. Given that, the explanations I read about for my leg problem made sense. With high hopes, I embarked on a series of daily exercises to strengthen my glutes. I also stopped running.

Though I felt better almost immediately, that didn't last. This approach acted like a placebo and contributed to short-term improvements, yet the pain came back a few weeks later as bad or worse than before. So, I saw an osteopath (also a functional medicine practitioner) who examined me, put me through a range of different motions, and told me nothing was physically wrong with my knee. But he noticed my hip was tight and could be the source of the pain lower down. He suggested getting a therapeutic massage.

The deep massage eased my pain, but it wasn't a cure. The masseur told me that, in my right hip, I had all the symptoms of bursitis, a chronic inflammation of the joint many people accept as a symptom of aging. He said that, in his experience, not much could be done to heal it. In fact, he said it commonly begins the familiar road toward getting a hip replacement.

At that point, the pain increased even more, especially in my knee. A friend noted that I was walking with a slight limp and my gait seemed stiff. Plus, it hurt to sit for long periods and hurt even more to stand up until I got moving again and my leg loosened up. Worry set in.

For the first time in four years, I had to miss the yearly thirty-mile springtime charity walk I do with my daughters up and down the hills of Oxfordshire. While I could still go to the gym and do various forms of exercise without trouble, getting out of bed or moving from a stationary position hurt, and I couldn't sleep on my right side.

Was this the start of my mobility being compromised? Would the pain gradually get worse until I needed a new knee, hip, or both? Still, I didn't want to consider a surgical option.

After only ten years, my plans to be fully functional had hit a major roadblock, and I wasn't even seventy years old. My quality of life depended on mobility, and that meant walking pain-free. Until then, I had taken the health and strength of my legs for granted—and I finally realized how precious the simple act of walking without discomfort was. Feeling much inner distress, I prayed and engaged whatever forces I could muster to find a solution.

Orthopedic Doctor's Counsel

Finally, I met with a recommended orthopedic doctor who specializes in sport injuries. Like the osteopath, his initial exam and ultrasound of my knee revealed nothing was wrong structurally. What a relief. However, a follow-up MRI of my knee showed a torn outer meniscus, the pad of cartilage in between the knee bones. At least that explained the knee pain, but he said he doubted this would cause my hip pain. To stabilize the region, he advised general strengthening of the legs and especially the glutes—similar to what I'd found in my web consultations.

He also said that fifteen or twenty years before, doctors would probably have operated on the meniscus to either repair or remove it. But now, and especially the way he practiced, he would recommend strengthening the area first. Bearing the complications from treatments ranging from cortisone injections to surgery weren't worth the risk. That meant seeing if physical rehab would be effective. I told him I was no stranger to hard work and would let him know what happened after doing strengthening exercises for my knee and hip. In response, he commented, "The problem is that most people who see me want a doctor to fix them and not to have to do anything to fix themselves." He was definitely *my* kind of doctor, and I was *his* kind of patient—someone committed to avoiding medical procedures and not afraid to put in the effort required.

For some, pills, shots, or surgery seem to confer magic to the healing process. But realistically, they involve more risk than trying to heal through natural means. *In the long run, I believe tampering with my body's ability to heal itself involves even more risk.*

I also had a follow-up session with a physiotherapist who admitted that many of her patients complain of pain yet there's no apparent medical cause. Privately, she agreed when I said their problems could have emotional sources. She said she knew practitioners who believe the same thing but don't admit it to patients for fear of losing their jobs or certification.

The Path That Worked

Increasingly focused on finding a solution, I tried massage, acupuncture, manipulation, classical exercise, and anti-inflammatory medication. All had no lasting effect, so I began thinking my condition might be psychosomatic. Perhaps hidden emotions were the source of different muscle tensions and imbalances that, in turn, caused my joints to function improperly. In *Heal Your Body A–Z*, Louise Hay wrote that hips are our center of moving forward in life and knees are the center of ego-related blockages. This made sense and certainly could apply to me—or at least provide a source for reflection.

I reread Dr. John Sarno's books at this time. In them, I found the area he associated with what I call the Sarno syndrome is the lower back, usually on one side or the other. Symptoms from this area involve being tense and contracted as a result of repressed inner anger and rage. *This was precisely what I was feeling.* He said this contraction, which I had experienced on and off during my life, can express itself in the hips, knees, and legs. He gave case studies of people with that diagnosis who experienced improvement after treatment and from understanding the inner dynamics. They also had greater control over any symptoms when they reappeared. All this happened without painkillers, anti-inflammatories, or surgery. The first step toward healing was to acknowledge that these buried emotions might be playing a part in my condition. In an even deeper way than when dealing with my bad back, I was open to the possibility that answers might lie in my subconscious. This increased my hope for a solution.

In the world of psychosomatic medicine, still in its infancy, Dr. Sarno's work represents a trusted and effective philosophy. He combines actual medical experience with an open mind and heart, plus the ability to understand the complexities of the integrated body. I view him as a true physician who ventured outside traditional medicine to help people relieve their suffering. Many MDs along my journey (including my first detox doctor and well-known ones like Dr. Mark Hyman and Dr. Andrew Weil) have also embraced a broader view of healing beyond conventional Western medicine. These range from diet and movement to emotional and spiritual paths, which align beautifully with my philosophy—*helping nature do the healing*.

Iyengar Yoga Teacher Comes to My Aid

Also on this path was my trusted friend and yoga teacher Nikki Costello. As serendipity would have it, at the time I told her about my leg pain, she said she'd just finished a therapeutic healing course at the Iyengar Institute in India. So, she worked with me to increase the strength of my hips and legs in ways I hadn't been able to do previously. The wonderful thing about yoga is its intricate ways of engaging subtle sensations, not only in the big muscle groups but in the small muscles, tendons, and nerves involved in rotation and balance. Minor muscle groups support the hips and knees and keep them aligned. Through age and/or lack of use, they lose their strength and flexibility, which leads to chronic inflammation and immobility.

Nikki had me do supported versions of three standard yoga poses:

triangle pose, warrior pose, and parsvakonasana or extended angle pose. I would go deep into the joints of both my right and left hips to strengthen muscles I didn't normally use. Trying to balance the muscle effort while relaxing other parts of my body was intense. In addition to strengthening my legs and hips, the poses increased blood circulation to the areas in ways regular exercise and physio had not. In turn, these postures helped promote the healing I was seeking, and I have been mostly pain-free ever since.

The Bottom Line—Daily Practice

Following this path took a few months of hard daily practice. Simultaneously, I worked on my inner self, reaffirming the importance of being able to walk for years to come. *I was worth the effort.* As the discomfort in my leg lessened, I could resume most of my regular activities with little or no pain. Nikki said it was not a permanent fix, but to retain and improve the joint stability I had achieved, I'd have to do this practice every day for the rest of my life.

"Every day for the rest of my life"—those were scary words. And she was right. If I take off more than a couple of days, I usually feel the discomfort again. Likewise, if I'm being particularly hard on myself or angry about something, pain sometimes presents itself in my hip or lower back. Caring for myself physically and emotionally— making the time and effort to heal—have become the mainstays of my therapeutic practice. Thankfully, the effort has become more enjoyable as I appreciate how my practice promotes health and helps me remain active and energetic.

The Underlying Remedy

My yoga remedy is one most people would identify with—that is, physical rehabilitation. But as difficult as the physical element can be, the psychological element is harder. As Dr. John Sarno writes: "You are experiencing the physical pain or symptom because it is easier and more acceptable to be in physical pain than coming to terms with the unconscious emotional truth that is the actual buried source."[1]

Realizing that physical symptoms have their origins in unconscious feelings has brought me relief and acceptance. The relief applies to common aches, pains, and upsets like headaches, digestive disorders, and persistent muscular problems. In addition to Dr. Sarno, I found the works of these authors relevant: Alice Miller in *The Body Never Lies*, Bessel van der Kolk in *The Body Keeps the Score*, and Gabor Maté in *The Myth of Normal*. These books have been friends to me as I heal my trauma-related physical symptoms. (See Bibliography.)

An Unexpected Bonus

People may not be aware that taking a *psychological* path to healing is possible. They simply say, "I'll get a shot of cortisone or, if I have to, I'll get my hip or knee replaced." Yet the self-engaged, holistic way I used ended up being more than a natural fix. The extra power and strength in my hips and legs proved to be a springboard to further positive changes. The more I practiced, the more I became conscious of my spine, which has taken the form of *feeling* my own posture. I began noticing the hunched-over appearance of people my age and the duck-like way they'd walk when their hips started to freeze. In that position, their posture is affecting their lungs, internal organs, and circulation. How could I prevent this in myself?

Becoming preoccupied with my spine was key. My goal was to increase the strength, flexibility, and "space" between the vertebrae in my spine. I hadn't even been aware of this because of the prior weakness in my hips. Then I started to focus on doing headstands, handstands, elbow stands, backbends, and other yoga poses to extend my spine. These poses make up a whole extra layer of my practice.

Full Breathing and Posture

One Sunday, I woke up early and lay in bed while my daughters slept. I started doing deep, controlled abdominal breathing—*pranayama* in yoga—to help my organs and digestive system awaken. A unique sensation happened that day—one I'd never experienced before. Rather than my in breath ending at the top of my lungs at neck level, I experienced the breath fully occupying not only my lungs but shooting up my spine and neck to the top of my head. This released my neck and shoulders into a deep relaxation on the exhale—a feeling I hadn't known until that point. For most of my life, this energy had been stopping at my collarbone and accumulating as neck and shoulder tension. But my breathing that day represented a giant awakening—a sensation of space, light, and energy in the form of increased blood flow to that area. This mirrored a vital energy pathway used by the fascia system and in yoga and acupuncture, as well as the connection between my brain and body.

That revelatory sensation hasn't left me. Friends say I stand straighter and seem taller than before. Changes in my body have resulted in my walking differently. I have become more conscious of all the elements involved in taking each step from head to toe. The result? An all-over gait that gently swings me back and forth with a slight twisting motion in my legs, hips, and spine. I stand with my feet slightly wider apart than before. My hips are not one-sided; they are more equally balanced than they were, and I feel better supported, more solid. My rib cage also feels better supported and hangs by my spine. The back of my body is as important as the front in supporting me. When I walk, I feel relaxed and engaged.

Hunching Over

This whole posture experience triggered a flood of associations from my childhood. As mentioned, I've always been tall. I was taller than my four-foot-ten mother by the time I was ten, and I towered over her by more than a foot by age sixteen. This made me conscious of "coming down to her level," which meant hunching over (literally and emotionally) to appease her. I wasn't "standing up for myself," so this desire to comply was mirrored in my posture.

Today, awareness of my posture as a way of standing, breathing, and being has become a part of my bones. At this age, I can finally *see* and *feel* the difference, and that has brought relief and insight. Emotionally, this awareness reinforced for me how deeply old currents run and how interconnected they are.

Tasty Fruits

At Christmas one year, our two-week family ski holiday to the Austrian Alps included my daughters, my ex-wife, and me complete with my newly rehabbed hip and knee. I hadn't skied in years, so I wore a right knee brace, recommended by the doctor for the torn meniscus. I fell a lot at first, yet eventually recovered some form and could negotiate the slopes with pleasure. My hips and legs were rock solid, stronger than I ever remembered them to be. Had I not pursued the rehab course I did, that ski trip would not have happened so wonderfully. I'd have been the old man sitting in the hotel instead of skiing with my family.

The following year, my eleven-year-old daughter Lollie and I completed the springtime thirty-mile charity walk, the one I couldn't do the previous year. For the first time, she finished the entire walk, proudly equaling her sister's record as the youngest ever to do so. I was thrilled to be with her and finish the walk myself. My knees and hips were again rock solid, albeit tired, but I had no pain, no lasting effects, and no reinjury. Both these experiences were tasty fruits of my committed journey toward longevity and vitality.

LESSON TWO: FIXING A BROKEN HEART

"What does the heart have to do with love? Probably nothing, according to your cardiologist . . . And yet, across centuries and across cultures, so many countless people—poets, writers, lovers, mothers, fathers, children, even scientists—have experienced love and connected it with the heart."

—DR. THOMAS COWAN, MD, *Human Heart, Cosmic Heart*

I began this book with an awakening about my life that involved my own father and the father I wanted to be to my daughters. The story of my heart problems and how I've learned to heal them represents a deeper dive into those dynamics. It spans several years on the medical front but ultimately goes back decades to my childhood. As the words above express, one's heart is about more than medical conditions. Although it doesn't possess the nerve density of the gut, which has the nickname "second brain," the heart is so sensitive to our inner emotional rhythms that it represents an interactive mirror of our being.

I've had two episodes of atrial flutter, an irregular heart rhythm similar to atrial fibrillation. This irregularity causes my heart to beat rapidly and stutter on the second part of the heartbeat. The first episode reverted to normal on its own after about six weeks. The second, which came eighteen months later, was fixed by a surgical procedure called a catheter ablation. I've also had a coronary scan that shows the beginnings of soft plaque buildup in one of my four heart arteries. To this, I can add a lifelong heart murmur, probably the result of undiagnosed rheumatic fever when I was a child. So, my heart has exhibited both electrical and circulatory weaknesses that needed attention. And finding the healing I needed to fix my "broken heart" has sharply illuminated my journey.

My Heart—First Episode

On the surface, too much caffeine provoked the first episode of atrial flutter on top of an over-the-counter decongestant I was taking for a cold. At least, that's what the cardiologist gave as a comfortable explanation. However, it occurred at a time of emotional upheaval for me. The doctors didn't want to hear about any emotional aspects, yet I suspected a link existed.

I experienced the first "flutter" as a nervousness in my chest as well as an extremely high heart rate I noticed in the gym. My heart was beating about 20 beats a minute *more* than my usual workout rates. I immediately went to a cardiologist who gave me an electrocardiogram and explained arrythmia to me. We scheduled a cardioversion, a noninvasive electric shock to the heart, to try and put my heart back into normal sinus rhythm. Because the condition elevates the risk of stroke, I took blood thinners for six weeks before the procedure.

To everyone's surprise, a week before the procedure was scheduled, my heart went back into a normal rhythm on its own. Yet, during that stretch of time, I was exploring other less traditional methods of relief in alignment with my diagnostic recipe: an osteopath, an acupuncturist, increased magnesium supplements, and increased work with my therapist. As counterintuitive as these links were in medical terms, what happened seemed to cohere.

I researched possible causes of my condition. Louise Hay's *Heal Your Body A–Z* stated that the heart is about love, and that *lack* of love can cause heart problems. This link felt right. In the meantime, my therapy work proved invaluable. My therapist said another patient with a similar condition had episodes of irregular heartbeat when she repressed her anger. I definitely felt angry with myself for having this condition at all—for needing to go through this process and not being healed and perfect without trying. I also had to endure the trials of self-discovery and felt frustrated that I wasn't yet cured of *my* emotional and physical baggage. Physical and emotional elements blurred. *What a turbulent time.*

This seemed similar to my John Sarno work, except that treating a heart was more serious than treating a bad back. In both cases, self-anger provided the fuel. Much of my anger had been subconscious. Earlier in life, I had expressed it more than my parents allowed, so I learned to suppress it. And now I was subconsciously angry with the circumstances and players from my past as well as with the emerging, vulnerable version of my present self.

During this time, I read *Human Heart, Cosmic Heart* by Thomas Cowan, MD, about his experience with arrhythmia and links he'd found to emotional causes. This work touched me and felt like the right path to pursue.

The night before my heartbeat reset itself naturally, I was at a cocktail party in New York, a rare activity since I had stopped drinking. Yet, I remember a different essence of me showed up there. I was not shy and withdrawn in the absence of drinking. Rather, I let me be myself as I talked with others about what mattered to me. I didn't have to please or confront these people, to make them laugh, strike a chord, agree, or disagree with them. If someone didn't understand what I was saying, the conversation soon drifted. But I didn't chastise myself when I couldn't explain myself well, and I didn't silently criticize them for not understanding, either. I had a sense of genuine social ease that brought forth good, casual conversations, nothing earth shaking. How different that felt from being at parties in the past! I simply let me *be myself* without putting on an act.

The following morning, I woke up relaxed and proud of how I'd felt the night before. My heart wasn't stuttering; it had reset itself to a normal sinus rhythm, one that lasted for a few days before I called my cardiologist. She was surprised at the news and skeptical, yet she confirmed it when I visited as she read the results of the electrocardiogram. My heart stayed in its "regular" rhythm for about another year and half.

My Heart—Second Episode

In the run-up to the second episode, big changes were happening inside—so much so that I had started drinking alcohol again a few months earlier. As before, drinking gave me a false sense of assurance that everything was okay. However, the sense of "me" I'd experienced at that New York party was gone, replaced by an old familiar bravado.

In retrospect, I realized I was trying to numb myself from something that needed to emerge. Around that time, I started working on a "life review"—a loose autobiography. I got this idea from Jane Fonda's *Prime Time* as well as from Natalie Goldberg and the uninhibited journal ramblings she advocates in *Writing Down the Bones*. Chronicling my life and seeing what unresolved issues came up could help me move forward. I was already journaling every morning, so I decided to focus that effort into a timeline of my life.

The day before the atrial flutter returned, I had been working on a passage that dealt with my father's death in 1957. This followed earlier entries about my adoption, my early childhood, my parents, their journey to America, and my young years in 1950s Newark, New Jersey. Here are excerpts from a longer original:

> In the early part of 1957, everything started to change ominously. My father went back into the hospital. The next thing I knew, my Uncle Max, my father's youngest brother came down from Montreal. I was told by my mother that I was going to go live in Montreal for a little while and go to school there. I can't remember the reason I was given. But I had no voice in the decision. It was decided for me, a fait-accompli dictate from her. I'm not sure I minded at first as I enjoyed spending time with my cousins so much. I couldn't process what a few months meant and was certainly not aware what awaited me in school there.
>
> The experience proved very frustrating. The Canadian school system emphasized different things in these early years, like cursive handwriting, gym, and French, all of which I had never had. They turned out not to be my strong suit. So, while I did OK in academics, I was struggling to make new friends and find any common ground with the other kids there. I felt like my support system had been ripped away and, other than the company I had in my new home with my aunt, uncle, and cousins, I desperately missed my family and my home.
>
> I remember getting very angry about all this while I was there, which was quite unlike the normally extremely well-behaved little boy I had become. Even though my mother later tried to explain to me that she was trying to protect me, I felt like I was being left out of MY family, that I had been dispatched somewhere else to be out of the way, that somehow,

I wasn't important enough or worthy enough to have around, that I was being excluded and that I didn't matter.

My time in Montreal lasted three months at which point my mother came to pick me up and bring me home. She told me that my father had died from his sickness. She explained what a big funeral he had and about how many people came to pay their respects and how well liked he was. Yet I had been denied being any part of this. I hadn't gotten to say goodbye to him.

There was more—how left out I felt, how unloved I felt, how distraught my mother was, and how I had to bury all my feelings. My life changed immeasurably when I lost my "best" parent and best friend, my dad. Feeling sidelined and ignored, I was often told how to behave by my mother. She was consumed by grief but never let me express mine. When she'd go into raging tantrums toward life and me, I had no one to turn to for support.

That night, after writing this section, I woke up feeling the familiar rapid heartbeat and stuttering sensation in my chest. The atrial flutter had returned. I wasn't as alarmed as the first time, thinking it would reset itself again. But it didn't.

After a few weeks, I went back to the cardiologists, this time consulting two of them to see if their opinions differed. Since it had happened twice, they both recommended a surgical procedure called an ablation. Again, there were physical reasons for it—my drinking (even in small amounts can trigger heart arrhythmias) and a high-intensity gym session the day before. The doctors were comfortable with these reasons, then added I was prone to this condition for some reason, genetic or otherwise. They hesitated to give any credence to emotional causes when I mentioned this. Yet, associating the flutter with my writing the morning before happened immediately. That truth had struck a deep chord. And the timing was too coincidental to ignore.

The Procedure

In the heat of doctors, hospitals, drugs, and surgery, it's easy to get overwhelmed and push everything else aside. Modern medicine holds this power over us. That day, I put my life in their hands. The ablation was done under general anesthesia in the morning, and I returned home later that evening. The operation was clinical, controlled, regulated, and monitored, with no room for speculation or insight. The doctors and surgeons, like airplane pilots, left nothing to chance, performing the procedure flawlessly. It's what Western medicine is best at: intervention and fixing. Yet once *their* work is done, even the medics must rely on the body's miraculous ability to recover from the trauma, however beneficial the surgery might be.

After this successful operation, my heart had a steady sinus rhythm. In a few weeks, I went back to regular activities, albeit cautiously. Even though the doctors pronounced me "fixed," I sensed that experiencing a complete recovery, both physically and emotionally, needed more time.

Care for My Heart

To find the best way to promote the well-being of my heart, I came at healing it from several directions. The conventional medical route was obvious: regular check-ups and monitoring of my heart by a trusted cardiologist. Yet medics rarely address the preventive and nonphysical aspects of health—the aspects that can't be measured. A regular electrocardiogram (ECG), blood pressure readings, and periodic blood tests for lipids and inflammation are their main tools. Add to that sonograms, stress tests, and CT scans, which I discuss below.

Subtle Battle

My heart deeply connects to my inner life, which goes back eons in evolution. The subtle balance among stress, electricity, and hormones is more than fight or flight, especially given the triggers for stress in modern life.

In my case, the *perceived* danger I felt as a child is rooted in emotions that still reside within me and can be triggered by present experiences. This contrasts to *actual* danger or fear for life and limb by, for example, being hit by a car. Part of the chronic stress people experience is this underground *perceived* variety. And given the constant physical stress of modern living, ill heart health can result.

The connection between my heart and the hurt from my childhood that surfaced in my journaling was too strong to ignore. My biological self was screaming, "Leave things alone. You can't feel these without endangering your survival." But my compassionate self was saying, "It's okay. You won't die; you need to feel these emotions now so you can grow and heal." My heart got caught in the middle. This unending journey through my childhood emotions has had many ups and downs. They've been the source of many joyous as well as painful moments in the present. Their negative effects have lessened with effort and time, and the benefits of my work have vastly increased the positive effects. As a result, my heart has been able to heal on several fronts.

Signs of a Healing Heart

Since the ablation procedure, I have religiously paid attention to my heart. My cardiologist was pleased that its rhythm has remained stable over the past six years. My resting heart rate has returned to around 55–60 beats a minute. I have resumed and even increased my previous high-intensity aerobic activities. A lingering wariness that persisted for a year or more has disappeared.

I'm ultrasensitive to caffeine and alcohol, so I've mostly stopped drinking both. Their physical effects—poor sleep, inflammation, low immune function, and lethargy—are loaded with emotional history and baggage. They remind me of a life I no longer want or need to live.

An Alarming CT Scan

About five years ago, I had a CT scan to see what's happening in the arteries of my heart. I have always had low LDL cholesterol and high HDL, so nothing amiss was expected. But what the scan revealed—a slight buildup of arterial plaque in one of my heart arteries—alarmed me. I had experienced no symptoms, and a follow-up stress test and sonogram yielded an extremely high 13.5 METs reading with no irregularities (a great result even for someone twenty years younger!). *How long had that plaque been present? Was it a recent development?* My cardiologist, who knows my health regime, told me that, for anyone else, she'd recommend a low-dose statin to reduce the LDL cholesterol. I declined that offer and have opted to 1) further reduce saturated fat in my diet, 2) maintain my already high levels of HIIT as well as my low-level aerobics, and 3) take a supplement of red yeast rice (with its natural version of statin medication).

Three years later, as my follow-up CT scan got closer, I realized how worried I had been about this appointment. What if it showed more plaque? I would have to take a statin and face all kinds of new medical monitoring to protect myself. I might have to slow down and reduce my level of activity. *This is NOT the way I wanted to spend my later years.*

The new scan results, though, showed no change in buildup and no evidence of any new plaque. In addition, my LDL cholesterol had gone down by 20 percent and my METs and VO$_2$ max levels were the same as the previous stress test. The cardiologist who had recommended a statin three years earlier told me she was "humbled" by these results. "Whatever you're doing is showing results better any conventional medical treatment," she said, adding I didn't need to see her again for a few years. My relief was palpable.

Unknowingly, I had been worrying about these results greatly. Learning that my heart was healthy produced an incredible boost in energy and spirit and reinforced my confidence that my health practices were on track.

The Heart: Organ of Love

Thomas Cowan writes in *Human Heart, Cosmic Heart* that the heart is not a pump. Therefore, no amount of "pump" physics can make the heart push hard enough for blood to make the full circulation through the body's arteries, capillaries, and veins. Rather, many energies and physics at play involve bodily systems and deeper rhythms. Ultimately, heart attacks and heart disease are caused by an imbalance between the sympathetic and parasympathetic nervous systems, which means the heart muscle doesn't "relax" enough in its parasympathetic resting phase. If it doesn't relax enough and accumulates too much lactic acid, the muscle becomes "hard-hearted," thus increasing the chances of artery blockage. This is especially true when our bodies are loaded down with too much saturated fat and sugar.

The factors that can cause this imbalance and poor circulation are many—from the stresses of modern life to not enough movement to poor diet to internal emotional issues including a lack of love. Dr. Cowan made the case that clogged arteries in themselves are not the sole cause of heart attacks and that it would be shortsighted to overlook the millennia-old association of our hearts with love.

Our hearts have also been associated with our souls. I affirm that I love my children with all my heart and soul, and now I can say *I love myself* more than ever, too. My grieving experiences have made me feel more wholehearted—more integrated and accepting of myself. All my practices have emerged as loving gifts to my heart in return for its ceaseless work of keeping me alive.

LESSON THREE: TICK, TICK, BAM!

In mid-August 2022, life was good on the North Fork of Long Island with my daughters and their friends enjoying our usual summer activities in and around the water—biking, eating, driving around, and just hanging out. I was feeling exceptionally strong and healthy, having boosted my exercise levels to new heights.

But one Friday afternoon, I came home from the gym feeling extremely tired. I also felt chilly despite the warm weather. My temperature was mildly elevated, about 99.5 degrees Fahrenheit or 37.5 Celsius. I suspected I had overdone it in the warm weather resulting in a mild heatstroke, so I took it easy that weekend.

But the fatigue didn't go away. I had the girls to take care of, so I struggled through the next ten days before they returned to England. From checking symptoms online, Lollie suspected Lyme disease, so I went to test for tickborne parasites or other systemic possibilities. (Deer and ticks are everywhere in Long Island, but they'd never been a problem for us.) The blood tests took a while, but the results confirmed I not only had Lyme disease but another tickborne disease called babesiosis. I began taking three different antibiotics and returned to New York City where I didn't have to drive and had more medical support. The doctor said it could take me as long as three weeks to recover.

Once my daughters left, I felt so weak, I couldn't stand up for more than thirty seconds. I had friends and grocery services supply me with food, but I had no appetite other than occasional cravings. After a week like this, my fever lingered, I lost weight, and I slept about twelve hours a day. My blood pressure dropped, mostly under 100/60. I packed a small bag just in case I had to go to the hospital.

And two mornings later, I felt so weak that I took a cab to the emergency room of my network hospital NYU Tisch. There, the doctors kept me for twenty-four hours and scheduled every test and procedure imaginable. Once again, I experienced the wonder and efficiency of modern medicine. The tests showed I had Lyme disease, babesiosis, *and* mononucleosis—all three at once. In addition to the fever and ultra-low blood pressure, I had low sodium levels and high inflammation levels, which they treated with drips and pills. This improved the situation enough for me to go home the next morning. The doctors told me to continue the antibiotics and anti-inflammatories, and they warned me to be patient. I planned to visit my primary care provider in a few weeks for a follow-up.

At the time of this writing, May 2023, it has been eight months since this hospital visit. When I first got home, I had no energy. It took six weeks of slow improvement, three of them on antibiotics, to have enough energy to leave my apartment and walk a couple of blocks. I had lost fifteen pounds and forced myself to eat despite still having no appetite. My friends and family stayed in constant touch out of worry and support. Gradually improving, I began stretching and doing easy yoga poses at home. Since then, I have ever so slowly gone back to the gym and gained strength and endurance. I feel 100 percent on most days. My immune system is gradually getting stronger and stronger, a testament to its indefatigable nature that I am reminded of every day. Until recently I lacked the stamina, strength, and surplus I had the previous summer. Now I am beginning to feel as healthy as I was then. Stay tuned . . .

The Path to Recovery

Neither by nature nor disposition am I a patient person. Part of my business acumen was getting things done quickly and efficiently. But recovering from my illness had a rhythm all its own, one I needed to follow rather than "make it happen." Healing is different for all of us. In my case, it's been a "two steps forward, one step back" pattern. Learning how to accept the one step back without seeing it as a disappointment has been a big benefit.

My life plan and priorities mentioned at the start of Part II have again become my beacon. Knowing *what I want*—health, vitality, joy, and longevity—gives me the energy and hope to stick with my recovery. I've learned that my joints, especially my knees, are weaker than before. That has led me to a physiotherapist whose program of weight-bearing exercise is making my knees stronger and more stable than before.

These setbacks have provided lessons on the role health problems play. In every case, those I've experienced are blessings because they showed me weaknesses that needed to be addressed. Whether it's my heart, my knees, my hips, or even the random contraction of Lyme disease, the exquisite sensory web within me knows my passion for life, so it brings problems to my attention. If they stayed in place, they would weaken me even further until the problems became chronic or unsolvable. That's not acceptable!

Yet Another Moment of Inspiration

While I had Lyme disease, I placed a chair halfway between the bedroom and the kitchen. I lacked the energy to walk the whole way at one time. I had to breathe and then rest. That made me aware that my inhale descended deeply into my abdomen and connected to the ultimate source of health and healing inside, the vital organs in my gut. I stayed with this slow abdominal breathing and felt this sensation for a while, keeping my mind empty and letting the connection flourish. This energy seemed as powerful (if not more powerful) as any prescription.

That moment provided me with a special resource—that is, whenever I don't feel well or feel anxious and afraid, I get in touch with this healing force simply by *breathing in* and *breathing out*. I breathe as deeply into the bottom of my abdomen as possible. This source of connection and safety is *always* part of me. As much as I can, I encourage this power to look after me, heal me, and inspire me.

CONCLUSION

Loving Life
The Endless Journey

"I celebrate myself, and sing myself,"
—WALT WHITMAN, Song of Myself

When I started this journey, I thought that the circumstances of my life—my job, my family, my wealth—were all that mattered. The universe woke me up and taught me an unending lesson, that the vast part of me *within* is bigger than my little ego self. And that inside part runs the show and connects to the world around me. It's what gives me energy and health.

I regret not having experienced this before, yet I'm exceedingly grateful to know it in my later years. The insight comes with vulnerability, sorrow, anxiety, and ambiguity as well as joy, gratitude, and ever-increasing knowledge of how "I" work. The world both within me and outside of me rumbles along to its evolving rhythms, and I'm happily along for the ride.

At age seventy-three, I have come to love life itself as well as the health it gives me. My daughters, ages nineteen and sixteen, are into their young adult lives, venturing into the never-ending journey of self-realization each person takes. My wish for them is to experience their own version of what I have learned for myself in recent years. My daughters still need my support but in very different ways than when they were children. I continue to feel grateful for the quality time I've had with them in their formative years and look forward to more of that precious time as their emerging lives allow.

Living life by the rules and for the wishes of others is the *safe* path, but living by your own inner voice is the *true* one. Again, you can't borrow life; you need to seek it out on your own terms and learn it anew for yourself.

THE VOICE OF LOVING LIFE

Other than my health practice and launching this book and its website, I have no big plans. "Nothing to do and nowhere to go" are my mantras. No more forced, compulsive behavior. Everyday life will make its presence felt. I will deal with its demands guided by the new light and freedom I've acquired. Life is still a bumpy road, but one I'm familiar with navigating. Writing helps me dig out what's inside me. Writing poetry and short fiction interests me, and so does communicating with others.

While working on the last chapters, I had an attack of annoying background chatter that went like this:

"What are you going to do now?"

"You don't even know if this book is any good."

"Who do you think you are writing a book like a big shot? You're too big for your britches. Think you're some sort of hot shot?"

"Whatever you do, don't get noticed. Don't stand out! Fit in!"

These voices from my past (many belonging to my mother) have been embedded deep in my psyche. While I can't silence them completely, I've learned either to ignore them or stand up against their dire forebodings and false information. Today, I have the wisdom to know that none of these voices are true, that I was treated unfairly as a child, and that the self-anger and criticism I feel are linked to those experiences.

Instead, I listen to another voice, a true voice, a guiding light that comes from a deep place within. It tells me to stick to this path and remain true to its callings as it says:

"Everything is and will be okay. You are loved simply by the experience of being alive. Take a breath and feel the power that comes with that love."

ENDNOTES

Chapter 2

[1] Michael Pollan, *In Defense of Food: An Eater's Manifesto* (New York: Penguin Press, 2008).

Chapter 5

[1] Steven Pressfield, *The War of Art: Break Through the Blocks and Win Your Inner Creative Battles* (New York: Warner Books, 2003).

Chapter 6

[1] BBC/Oxford University, *The Placebo Experiment: Can My Brain Cure My Body?* presented by Dr. Michael Mosley, October 4, 2018, https://www.dailymotion.com/video/x6vbq52.

Chapter 7

[1] Mary Oliver, *Blue Pastures* (New York: Ecco, 1995).

Chapter 9

[1] Heinrich Zimmer, Joseph Campbell, ed., "The Roar of Awakening," *Philosophies of India* (Princeton, NJ: Princeton University Press, 1969), 2, "We can't borrow God. We must effect His new incarnation from within ourselves. Divinity must descend, somehow, into the matter of our own existence and participate in this peculiar life-process."

Part II

[1] Howard S. Friedman and Leslie R. Martin, *The Longevity Project: Surprising Discoveries for Health and Long Life from the Landmark Eight-Decade Study* (New York: Plume, 2012).

Chapter 11

[1] Herman Pontzer, "The Exercise Paradox," *Scientific American*, Feb. 1, 2017, https://www.scientificamerican.com/article/the-exercise-paradox/.

[2] Valter Longo, *The Longevity Diet: Discover the New Science Behind Stem Cell Activation and Regeneration to Slow Aging, Fight Disease, and Optimize Weight* (New York: Avery, 2018).

[3] Terry Wahls and Eve Adamson, *The Wahls Protocol: A Radical New Way to Treat All Chronic Autoimmune Conditions Using Paleo Principles* (New York: Avery, 2014).

[4] Valter Longo, *The Longevity Diet: Discover the New Science Behind Stem Cell Activation and Regeneration to Slow Aging, Fight Disease, and Optimize Weight* (New York: Avery, 2018).

Chapter 14

[1] Matthew Walker, *Why We Sleep: Unlocking the Power of Sleep and Dreams* (New York: Scribner, 2017).

Chapter 17

[1] Allen Wheelis, *How People Change* (New York: William Morrow, 1975).

Chapter 18

[1] Avery Posey, Carl June, Bruce Levine, "A New Model for Defeating Cancer: CAR T Cells," *Scientific American*, March 1,

2017, https://www.scientificamerican.com/article/a-new-model-for-defeating-cancer-car-t-cells/.

Chapter 21
[1] John E. Sarno, *The Mindbody Prescription: Healing the Body, Healing the Pain* (New York: Warner Books, 1999).

RESOURCES

Studies come in all shapes and sizes, from peer-reviewed scientific ones to others that become media and popular talking points. These ubiquitous reports can lead to information overload, particularly when presented as evidence to "prove" something, give advice, or sell a product. This is subjective territory.

I am not a scientist or a doctor; I have simply sought helpful information to further my longevity mission. What matters most is if a study makes sense to me and the author strikes a chord inside that says, "This might be worth seeing if it actually works." But the proof is in the pudding—my practice and how I respond to it—not in the often conflicting and self-serving evidence of popular studies.

Following are just a few of the many studies, books, programs, and documentaries that have "moved the needle" for me and, in addition to my selected bibliography, presented information that has made the most sense on my journey. From these suggestions, see what works for you!

STUDIES AND BOOKS CITED IN THIS BOOK

Amaral-Phillips, Donna M. "Are Your Dairy Cows Getting the Protein They Need?" University of Kansas Department and Food Sciences. Accessed July 19, 2023. https://afs.ca.uky.edu/files/are_your_dairy_cows_getting_the_protein_they_need.pdf.

Ames, Bruce N. "Increasing Longevity by Tuning Up Metabolism. To Maximize Human Health and Lifespan, Scientists Must Abandon Outdated Models of Micronutrients. " *European Molecular Biology Organization* 6 Suppl. 1 (July 2005): S20–S24. doi: 10.1038/sj.embor.7400426.

Ames, Bruce N. "Low Micronutrient Intake May Accelerate the Degenerative Diseases of Aging Through Allocation of Scarce Micronutrients by Triage." *Proceedings of the Nation Academy of Sciences* 103, no. 47 (November 21, 2006): 17589–94. doi: 10.1073/pnas.0608757103.

Atakan, Muhammed M., Yanchun Li, Nazan S. Koşar, and Huseyin Husrev Turnagol. "Evidence-Based Effects of High-Intensity Interval Training on Exercise Capacity and Health: A Review with Historical Perspective." *International Journal of Environmental Research and Public Health* 21, no. 13 (July 2021): 1–28. DOI:10.3390/ijerph18137201.

Berk, Michael, Lana J. Williams, Felice N. Jacka, Adrienne O'Neil, Julie A. Pasco, Steven Moylan, and Nicholas B. Allen. "So Depression Is an Inflammatory Disease, But Where Does the Inflammation

Come From?" *BMC Medicine* 11, no. 200 (September 12, 2013). doi: 10.1186/1741-7015-11-200.

Bredesen, Dale E., Edwin C. Amos, Jonathan Canick, Mary Ackerley, Cyrus Raji, Milan Fiala, and Jamila Ahdidane. "Reversal of Cognitive Decline in Alzheimer's Disease." *Aging* 8, no. 6 (June 2016): 1250–58. doi: 10.18632/aging.100981.

Catlin, George. *Letters and Notes on the Manners, Customs, and Condition of North American Indians*. New York: Dover, 1971.

Civitarese, Anthony E., Stacy Carling, Leonie K. Heilbronn, Mathew H. Hulver, Barbara Ukropcova, Walter A. Deutsch, Steven R. Smith, Eric Ravussin, and CALERIE Pennington Team. "Calorie Restriction Increases Muscle Mitochondrial Biogenesis in Health Humans." *Public Library of Science* 4, no. 3 (March 2007): e76. doi: 10.1371/journal.pmed.0040076.

Cutler, David M., Edward Glaeser, and Jesse Shapiro. "Why Have Americans Become More Obese?" Harvard Institute of Economic Research Working Paper No. 1994. January 23, 2003. https://papers.ssrn.com/sol3/papers.cfm?abstract_id=373121.

de Koning, Lawrence, Teresa T. Fung, Xiaomei Liao, Stephanie E. Chiuve, Eric B. Rimm, Walter C. Willett, Donna Spiegelman, and Frank B. Hu. "Low Carbohydrate Diet Scores and Risk of Type 2 Diabetes in Men." *American Journal of Clinical Nutrition* 93, no. 4 (April 2011): 844–50. doi: 10.3945/ajcn.110.004333.

Estruch, Ramón, Emilio Ros, Jordi Salas-Salvadó, Maria-Isabel Covas, Dolores Corella, Fernando Arós, Enrique Gómez-Gracia et al. "Primary Prevention of Cardiovascular Disease with a Mediterranean Diet." *New England Journal of Medicine* 368 (April 4, 2013): 1279–1290. DOI: 10.1056/NEJMoa1200303.

Fontana, Luigi. "Excessive Adiposity, Calorie Restriction, and Aging."

Journal of the American Medical Association 295, no. 13 (April 5, 2006): 1577–8. doi: 10.1001/jama.295.13.1577.

Fontana, Luigi, Linda Partridge, and Valter D Longo, "Extending Healthy Life Span—from Yeast to Humans." *Science* 328, no. 5976 (April 16, 2010). doi: 10.1126/science.1172539.

Fung, Teresa, Rob M. van Dam, Susan E. Hankinson, Meir Stampfer, Walter C. Willett, and Frank B. Hu. "Low Carbohydrate Diets and All-Cause and Cause-Specific Mortality: Two Cohort Studies." *Annals of Internal Medicine* 153, no. 5 (September 7, 2010): 289–98. doi: 10.7326/0003-4819-153-5-201009070-00003.

Gebel, Klaus, Ding Ding, Tien Chey, Emmanuel Stamatakis, Wendy J. Brown, and Adrian E. Bauman. "Effect of Moderate to Vigorous Physical Activity on All-Cause Mortality in Middle Aged and Older Australians." *JAMA Internal Medicine* 175, no. 6 (2015): 970–977. doi:10.1001/jamainternmed.2015.0541.

Gillen, Jenna B., Brian J. Martin, Martin J. MacInnis, Lauren E. Skelly, Mark A. Tarnopolsky, and Martin J. Gibala. "Twelve Weeks of Sprint Interval Training Improves Indices of Cardiometabolic Health Similar to Traditional Endurance Training Despite a Five-Fold Lower Exercise Volume and Time Commitment." *Public Library of Science (PLoS One)* 11, no. 4 (April 26, 2016): e0154075. doi: 10.1371/journal.pone.0154075.

Heilbronn, Leonie K., Lilian de Jonge, Madlyn I. Frisard, James P. DeLany, D. Enette Larson-Meyer, Jennifer Rood, Tuong Nguyen et al. "Effect of 6-Month Calorie Restriction on Biomarkers of Longevity, Metabolic Adaptation, and Oxidative Stress in Overweight Individuals." *Journal of the American Medical Association* 295, no. 13 (April 5, 2006): 1539–48. doi: 10.1001/jama.295.13.1539.

John Rae's Arctic Correspondence, 1844–1855. Hudson's Bay Record

Society. https://www.google.com/books/edition/John_Rae_s_Arctic_Correspondence_1844_18/V5klBAAAQBAJ?hl=en&gbpv=1.

Kossoff, Eric. "Ketogenic Diets in Seizure Control and Neurologic Disorders," in *The Art and Science of Low Carbohydrate Performance* (Beyond Obesity, 2012).

Longo, Valter. *The Longevity Diet*, Chapter 4. "Calorie Restriction: Mice, Monkeys, and Humans." New York: Avery, 2018.

Longo, Valter. *The Longevity Diet*, Chapter 7. "Nutrition and Fasting Mimicking Diets in Cancer Prevention and Treatment." New York: Avery, 2018. (This book is for general discussion of low carbohydrate, calorie reduction, and fasting.)

Manor, Ohad, Chengzhen L. Dai, Sergey A. Kornilov, Brett Smith, Nathan D. Price, Jennifer C. Lovejoy, Sean M. Gibbons, and Andrew T. Magis. "Health and Disease Markers Correlate with Gut Microbiome Composition Across Thousands of People." *Nature Communications* 11, no. 1 (October 15, 2020): 5206. doi: 10.1038/s41467-020-18871-1.

McCay, C. M., Mary F. Crowell, and L. A. Maynard. "The Effect of Retarded Growth upon the Length of Life Span and upon the Ultimate Body Size." *Journal of Nutrition* 10, no. 1 (July 1935): 63–79. https://doi.org/10.1093/jn/10.1.63. (First landmark study showing that calorie-restriction without malnutrition extends life span in rats.)

Meyer, Timothy E., Sándor J. Kovács, Ali A. Ehsani, Samuel Klein, John O. Holloszy, and Luigi Fontana. "Long Term Caloric Restriction Ameliorates the Decline in Diastolic Function in Humans," *Journal of the American College of Cardiology* 47, no. 2 (January 2006). https://www.jacc.org/doi/10.1016/j.jacc.2005.08.069.

O'Dea, Kerin. "Marked Improvement in Carbohydrate and Lipid Metabolism in 8/10/23 Diabetic Australian Aborigines After

Temporary Reversion to Traditional Lifestyle." *Diabetes* 33, no. 6 (June 1984): 596–603. doi: 10.2337/diab.33.6.596.

Orr, J.B. and J.L. Gilks. "Studies of Nutrition: The Physique and Health of Two African Tribes." *Medical Research Council*, London, 1935. https://searchworks.stanford.edu/view/13486666.

Psihoyos, Louie, dir. *The Game Changers*. Netflix (2018).

Russel, Jenni. "Fasting Transformed Me After Medicine Failed." *Times of London* (April 23, 2015). https://www.thetimes.co.uk/article/fasting-transformed-me-after-medicine-failed-rdxqr553hz0.

Sharma, Ashish, Vishal Madaan, and Frederick D Petty. "Exercise for Mental Health." *Journal of Clinical Psychiatry* 8, no. 2 (2006): 106. doi: 10.4088/pcc.v08n0208a.

Sharon, Gil, Nikki Jamie Cruz, Dae-Wook Kang, Michael J. Gandal, Bo Wang, Young-Mo Kim, Erika M. Zink et al. "Human Gut Microbiota from Autism Spectrum Disorder Promote Behavioral Symptoms in Mice." *CELL* 177, no. 6 (May 30, 2019): 1600–1618.e17. doi: 10.1016/j.cell.2019.05.004.

Spurlock, Morgan. *Super Size Me*. Samuel Goldwyn Films (2004).

Srikanthan, Preethi and Arun S. Karlamangla. "Muscle Mass Index as Predictor of Longevity." *American Journal of Medicine* 127, no. 6 (June 2014): 547–53. doi: 10.1016/j.amjmed.2014.02.007.

Stefansson, Vilhjalmur. *The Friendly Arctic*. New York: Macmillan, 1921.

Taubes, Gary. *Good Calories, Bad Calories: Fats, Carbs, and the Controversial Science of Diet and Health*. New York: Anchor, 2008. Especially chapter 5, "The Diseases of Civilization." (See Selected Bibliography as general lower carbohydrate advocate.)

Taubes, Gary. *Why We Get Fat: And What to do About It*. New York: Anchor, 2011.

"The Therapeutic and Preventive Potential of the Hunter-Gatherer

Lifestyle: Insights from Australian Aborigines" in *Western Diseases: Their Dietary Prevention and Reversibility*. Totowa, NJ: Humana Press, 2012.

Wahls, Terry. *The Wahls Protocol: A Radical New Way to Treat all Chronic Autoimmune Conditions Using Paleo Principles*. New York: Avery, 2014.

Willcox, Bradley J. D. Craig Willcox, and Makoto Suzuki. *The Okinawa Program: How the World's Longest-Lived People Achieve Everlasting Health—And How You Can Too*. New York: Harmony, 2002.

(also see Selected Bibliography)

B.K.S. IYENGAR TEN TIPS FOR A LONG AND HEALTHY LIFE

1. Breathe as if you are divine.
2. Health is the gateway to spiritual well-being.
3. Go inward.
4. Connect to something greater than yourself.
5. Strive for truth.
6. Embrace change.
7. Be willing to evolve.
8. Be patient with your practice.
9. On your birthday do as many backbends as you are years old.
10. Rest five minutes for every thirty minutes of practice.

ANNUAL BLOOD TESTS FOR HEALTH AND LONGEVITY (MEN)

25-hydroxy vitamin D

Apoplipoprotein A-1

Apoplipoprotein A-2

Blood lead

Blood mercury

Cardio IQ lipoprotein fractionation, ion mobility

Complete blood count w/ differential

Complete metabolic panel

Copper

Cortisol

Dehydroepiandrosterone sulphate

Estradiol

Ferritin, serum

Fibrinogen

Folate

Free fatty acids

HCrp

Hemoglobin A1C

Homocysteine

IGF-1 (Growth hormone surrogate)

Insulin

Iron, TIBC

Lipid panel

Lipoprotein (a)
Lipoprotein-associated phospholipase A2 (PLAC 2)
Luteinizing hormone
Omega-3 fatty acids
RBC magnesium
Reverse T-3
Selenium
SHBG (sex hormone binding globulin)
T-3 free
T-3 total
T-3 uptake
T-4 free
T-4 (thyroxine)
Testosterone + free testosterone
Thiamine
Thyroglobulin antibodies
Thyroid peroxidase AB
TSH
Uric acid
Vitamin A
Vitamin B12
Zinc

ADDITIONAL METABOLIC AND SUPPLEMENT TESTS

I suggest getting a food allergen cellular test, which is needed only once. Also, every few years, test for levels of these substances in your body:

Alpha-lipoic acid
Amino acid panel
Biotin—B7
Cobalamin—B12
CoEnzyme Q10
Fatty acid panel
Folic Acid—B9
Magnesium
Manganese
Molybdenum
Metabolic analysis panel
Niacin—B3
Oxidative stress markers
Pyridoxine—B6
Riboflavin—B2
Thiamin—B1
Toxic element panel
Vitamin A
Vitamin C
Vitamin D
Vitamin E/tocopherols
Zinc

CONSULTANT SOURCES

Some of my main regular sources of health, longevity, and matters of mind and spirit:

Dr. Mark Hyman
Ben Greenfield
Examine.com
Harvard Medical School (www.health.Harvard.edu)
Dr. Frank Lipman
Dr. Jeff Bland
Max Lugavere
The Marginalian by Maria Popova; themarginalian.org
Fight Aging (www.fightaging.org)
Public Library of Science (PLoS)
News sources:
    The New York Times
    BBC
    The Guardian
    Scientific American

SELECTED BIBLIOGRAPHY

Agus, David B. *The End of Illness.* New York: Simon & Schuster, 2012.

Agus, David B. *A Short Guide to a Long Life.* New York: Simon & Schuster, 2014.

Beare, Sally. *50 Secrets of the World's Longest Living People.* New York: Hatchette, 2009.

Biss, Eula. *On Immunity: An Inoculation.* Minneapolis, MN: Graywolf Press, 2014.

Bland, Jeffrey S. *The Disease Delusion: Conquering the Causes of Chronic Illness for a Healthier, Longer, and Happier Life.* New York: Harper, 2014.

Boorstein, Sylvia. *Don't Just Do Something, Sit There: A Mindfulness Retreat with Sylvia Boorstein.* New York: Harper, 1996.

Boorstein, Sylvia. *Happiness Is an Inside Job: Practicing for a Joyful Life.* New York: Ballantine, 2008.

Bowman, Katy. *Dynamic Aging: Simple Exercises for Whole-body Mobility.* Propriometrics Press, 2017.

Bowman, Katy. *Move Your DNA: Restore Your Health through Natural Movement.* Propriometrics Press, 2017.

Bowman, Katy *Movement Matters: Essays on Movement Science, Movement Ecology, and the Nature of Movement.* Propriometrics Press, 2016.

Brown, Brené. *Daring Greatly: How the Courage to be Vulnerable Transforms the Way We Live, Love, Parent, and Lead.* New York: Avery, 2015.

Brown, Stuart. *Play: How It Shapes the Brain, Opens the Imagination, and Invigorates the Soul*. New York: Avery, 2009.

Bryson, Bill. *The Body: A Guide for Occupants*. New York: Doubleday, 2019.

Bucke, Richard Maurice. *Cosmic Consciousness: A Study in the Evolution of the Human Mind*. White Crow Books, 2011.

Buettner, Dan. *The Blue Zones: Lessons for Living Longer from the People Who've Lived the Longest*. Washington, DC: National Geographic Society, 2010.

Cain, Susan. *Quiet: The Power of Introverts in a World That Can't Stop Talking*. New York: Crown, 2013.

Campbell, Joseph. *The Hero with a Thousand Faces*. Novato, CA: New World Library, 2008.

Campbell, Joseph. *Historical Atlas of World Mythology*, Volumes 1, 2, 3, and 4. New York: HarperCollins, 1988.

Campbell, Joseph. *The Inner Reaches of Outer Space: Metaphor as Myth and as Religion*. Novato, CA: New World Library, 2012.

Campbell, Joseph. *The Masks of God*, Volumes 1, 2, 3, and 4. New York: Penguin Books, 1976.

Campbell, Joseph. *The Mythic Dimension*. Novato, CA: New World Library, 1997.

Campbell, Joseph. *The Mythic Dimension: Selected Essays 1959–1987*. Novato, CA: New World Library, 2007.

Campbell, Joseph. *Myths to Live By*. New York: Penguin, 1993.

Campbell, Joseph and Bill Moyers. *The Power of Myth*. New York: Anchor Books, 1991.

Carpenter, Edward. *The Art of Creation: Essays on the Self and Its Powers*. 1904. https://archive.org/details/artcreationessa01carpgoog.

Carpenter, Edward. *Towards Democracy*. United States: BiblioBazaar, 2015.

Carr, Allen. *The Easy Way to Stop Drinking.* New York: Sterling Publishing Company, 2005.

Carr, Kris. *Crazy, Sexy Cancer Tips.* Tantor & Blackstone: 2019.

Chatterjee, Rangan. *How to Make Disease Disappear.* New York: HarperOne, 2018.

Cowan, Thomas. *Human Heart, Cosmic Heart: A Doctor's Quest to Understand, Treat, and Prevent Cardiovascular Disease.* Chelsea, VT: Chelsea Green Publishing, 2016.

Crowley, Chris and Henry S. Lodge. *Younger Next Year: Live Strong, Fit, and Sexy—Until You're 80 and Beyond.* New York: Workman, 2007.

Czerski, Helen. *Storm in a Teacup: The Physics of Everyday Life.* New York: W. W. Norton, 2017.

Dante Alighieri. *The Divine Comedy.* (Trans. By J. Ciardi). New York: Signet, 2003.

Dante Alighieri. *The Divine Comedy.* (Trans. By H. W. Longfellow). New York: Vintage, 1994.

Diamond, Jared. *Guns, Germs and Steel: The Fates of Human Societies.* New York: W. W. Norton, 1999.

Diamond, Jared. *The World Until Yesterday: What Can We Learn from Traditional Societies?* New York: Penguin, 2013.

Dubos, René. (1998). *A God Within: A Positive View of Mankind's Future.* New York: Scribners, 1972.

Dubos, René. *The Mirage of Health: Utopias, Progress, and Biological Change.* Rutgers, NJ: Rutgers University Press, 1987.

Dychtwald, Ken. *Bodymind: The Whole-Person Health Book: A Guide to Staying Well and Living Longer.* New York: Tarcher Putnam, 1986.

Fonda, Jane. *Prime Time: Love, Health, Sex, Fitness, Friendship, Spirit; Making the Most of All of Your Life.* New York: Random House, 2011.

Frankl, Viktor E. *Man's Search for Meaning*. New York: Pocket Books, 1985.

Frankl, Viktor E. *Man's Search for Ultimate Meaning*. New York: Basic Books, 2018.

Friedman, Howard S. and Leslie R. Martin, *The Longevity Project: Surprising Discoveries for Health and Long Life from the Landmark Eight-decade Study*. New York: Plume, 2012.

Fuhrman, Joel. *Eat to Live: The Amazing Nutrient-Rich Program for Fast and Sustained Weight Loss*. New York: Little, Brown, 2011.

García, Héctor and Francesc Miralles. *Ikigai: The Japanese Secret to a Long and Happy Life*. New York: Penguin, 2017.

Gawande, Atul. *Being Mortal*. New York: Metropolitan, 2017.

Gladwell, Malcolm. *Blink: The Power of Thinking Without Thinking*. New York: Back Bay, 2007.

Gladwell, Malcolm. *The Tipping Point: How Little Things Can Make a Big Difference*. New York: Little, Brown, 2006.

Godfred, Melody. *Self Love Poetry: For Thinkers and Feelers*. Andrews McMeel, 2021.

Godwin, Robert. *One Cosmos Under God: The Unification of Matter, Life, Mind, and Spirit*. Berkeley, CA: Paragon House, 2004.

Goldberg, Natalie. *Writing Down the Bones: Freeing the Writer Within*. Boulder, CO: Shambhala Publications, 1986.

Graeber, David and David Wengrow. *The Dawn of Everything: A New History of Humanity*. New York: Farrar, Straus and Giroux, 2021.

Greenfield, Ben. *Beyond Training: Mastering Endurance, Health, and Life*. Las Vegas: Victory Belt, 2014.

Grierson, Bruce. *What Makes Olga Run?: The Mystery of the 90-something Track Star and What She Can Teach Us About Living Longer, Happier Lives*. New York: St. Martin's Griffin, 2015.

Hanh, Thich Nhat. *The Art of Living: Peace and Freedom in the Here and Now.* New York: HarperOne, 2017.

Hanh, Thich Nhat. *How to Connect.* Berkeley, CA: Parallax Press, 2020.

Hanh, Thich Nhat. *How to Focus.* Berkeley, CA: Parallax Press, 2022.

Hanh, Thich Nhat. *How to Relax.* Berkeley, CA: Parallax Press, 2015.

Hanh, Thich Nhat. *Nothing to Do, Nowhere to Go: Reflections on the Teachings of Zen Master Lin Chi.* Berkeley, CA: Parallax Press, 2007.

Hay, Louise. *Heal Your Body A–Z: The Mental Causes for Physical Illness and the Way to Overcome Them.* Carlsbad, CA: Hay House, 1998.

Hay, Louise. *You Can Heal Your Life.* Carlsbad, CA: Hay House, 1984.

Hesse, Hermann. *The Seasons of the Soul: The Poetic Guidance and Spiritual Wisdom of Hermann Hesse.* Berkeley, CA: North Atlantic Books, 2011.

Hesse, Hermann. *Siddhartha.* New York: Penguin, 2002.

Heying, Heather and Bret Weinstein. *A Hunter-Gatherer's Guide to the 21st Century: Evolution and the Challenges of Modern Life.* New York: Portfolio, 2021.

Holford, Patrick and Jerome Burne. *The 10 Secrets of Healthy Aging: How to Live Longer, Look Younger, and Feel Great.* New York: Piatkus, 2012.

Horney, Karen. *Neurosis and Human Growth: The Struggle Toward Self-Realization.* New York: W. W. Norton, 1991.

Howard, Vernon. *The Mystic Masters Speak! A Treasury of Cosmic Wisdom.* New Life Foundation, 1988.

Huang, Alfred, translator. *The Complete I Ching.* Rochester, VT: Inner Traditions, 2010.

Hyman, Mark. *The Blood Sugar Solution: The Ultrahealthy Program for Losing Weight, Preventing Disease, and Feeling Great Now!* New York: Little, Brown, 2014.

Selected Bibliography

Hyman, Mark. *Eat Fat, Get Thin: Why the Fat We Eat Is the Key to Sustained Weight Loss and Vibrant Health.* New York: Little, Brown, 2016.

Hyman, Mark. *Food Fix: How to Save Our Health, Our Economy, Our Communities, and Our Planet—One Bite at a Time.* New York: Little, Brown, 2020.

Iyengar, B. K. S. *Light on Life: The Yoga Journey to Wholeness, Inner Peace, and Ultimate Freedom.* New York: Rodale, 2006.

Iyengar, B. K. S. *Light on Yoga: The Bible of Modern Yoga.* New York: HarperCollins, 2015.

Iyengar, B. K. S. *YOGA, the Path to Holistic Health.* New York: Dorling Kindersley, 2001.

Jung, C. G. *The Archetypes and the Collective Unconscious.* Princeton, NJ: Princeton University Press, 1981.

Junger, Alejandro. *Clean: The Revolutionary Program to Restore the Body's Natural Ability to Heal Itself.* New York: HarperOne, 2009.

Karen, Robert. *The Forgiving Self: The Road from Resentment to Connection.* New York: Anchor, 2003.

Katagiri, Dainin. *Returning to Silence: Zen Practice in Daily Life.* Boulder, CO: Shambhala Publications, 1988.

Katagiri, Dainin. *You Have to Say Something: Manifesting Zen Insight.* Boulder, CO: Shambhala Publications, 2000.

Kelly, Rachel. *Black Rainbow.* New York: Hodder & Stoughton, 2015.

Klein, Daniel. *Every Time I Find the Meaning of Life, They Change It.* New York: Penguin, 2017.

Klein, Daniel. *Travels with Epicurus: A Journey to a Greek Island in Search of a Fulfilled Life.* New York: Penguin, 2014.

Kresser, Chris. *Unconventional Medicine.* Lioncrest, 2017.

Lagakos, William. *The Poor, Misunderstood Calorie.* CreateSpace, 2012.

Lamott, Anne. *Bird by Bird: Some Instructions on Writing and Life.* New York: Knopf Doubleday, 1995.

Lamott, Anne. *Help, Thanks, Wow: The Three Essential Prayers*. New York: Riverhead, 2012.

Leach, Jeff D. *Rewild: Discovering the Art of Returning to Nature*. CreateSpace, 2015.

Levitin, Daniel J. *Successful Aging: A Neuroscientist Explores the Power and Potential of Our Lives*. New York: Dutton, 2020.

Lieberman, Daniel. E. *The Story of the Human Body: Evolution, Health, and Disease*. New York: Vintage, 2014.

Lipman, Frank. *The New Rules of Aging Well: A Simple Program for Immune Resilience, Strength, and Vitality*. New York: Artisan, 2020.

Longo, Valter. *The Longevity Diet: Discover the New Science Behind Stem Cell Activation and Regeneration to Slow Aging, Fight Disease, and Optimize Weight*. New York: Avery, 2018.

Lugavere, Max and Paul Grewal. *Genius Foods: Become Smarter, Happier, and More Productive While Protecting Your Brain for Life*. New York: Harper Wave, 2018.

Manson, Mark. *The Subtle Art of Not Giving a F*ck*. New York: Harper, 2016.

Marchant, Jo. *Cure: A Journey into the Science of Mind Over Body*. New York: Crown, 2017.

Maté, Gabor. *The Myth of Normal: Trauma, Illness and Healing in a Toxic Culture*. New York: Avery, 2022.

McGonigal, Kelly. *The Joy of Movement*. New York: Avery, 2021.

McGonigal, Kelly. *The Upside of Stress: Why Stress Is Good For You and How to Get Good at It*. New York: Avery, 2016.

McKeown, Patrick. *The Oxygen Advantage: The Simple, Scientifically Proven Breathing Techniques for a Healthier, Slimmer, Faster, and Fitter You*. New York: William Morrow, 2016.

Mehta, Silva, Mira Mehta, and Shyam Mehta. *Yoga, The Iyengar Way*. New York: Knopf, 2005.

Merton, Thomas. *Zen and the Birds of Appetite.* New York: New Directions, 1968.
Midgley, Mary. *Beast and Man: The Roots of Human Nature.* United Kingdom: Routledge, 2002.
Midgley, Mary. *Evolution as a Religion: Strange Hopes and Stranger Fears.* United Kingdom, Routledge, 2002.
Midgley, Mary. *The Myths We Live By.* United Kingdom: Routledge, 2011.
Miller, Alice. *The Body Never Lies: The Lingering Effects of Hurtful Parenting.* New York: W. W. Norton, 2006.
Miller, Alice. *The Drama of the Gifted Child: The Search for the True Self* (3rd ed.). New York: Basic Books, 1997.
Miller, Alice. *For Your Own Good: Hidden Cruelty in Child-Rearing and the Roots of Violence.* New York: Farrar, Strauss & Giroux, 1990.
Moore, Thomas. *Care of the Soul: A Guide for Cultivating Depth and Sacredness in Everyday Life.* New York: Harper, 2016.
Myers, Thomas. W. *Anatomy Trains: Myofascial Meridians for Manual and Movement Therapists.* New York: Elsevier, 2020.
Myss, Caroline. *Why People Don't Heal and How They Can.* New York: Harmony, 1998.
Needleman, Jacob. *I Am Not I.* Berkeley, CA: North Atlantic Books, 2016.
Nestor, James. *Breath: The New Science of a Lost Art.* New York: Riverhead Books, 2020.
Nuland, Sherwin. B. *How We Die: Reflections on Life's Final Chapter.* New York: Vintage, 1997.
Nurse, Paul. *What Is Life?* New York: W. W. Norton, 2021.
Oliver, Mary. *Blue Pastures.* New York: Ecco, 1995.
Oliver, Mary. *Devotions: Selected Poems.* New York: Penguin, 2017.
Oliver, Mary. *Upstream, Selected Essays.* New York: Penguin, 2016.

Oliver, Mary. *A Thousand Mornings, Poems*, New York: Penguin, 2013.

Oparin, A. I. *The Origin of Life.* Moscow: Foreign Language Publishing, 1955, https://archive.org/details/oparin-the-origin-of-life/mode/2up.

Osbon, Diane K., ed. *A Joseph Campbell Companion, Reflections on the Art of Living.* New York: Harper, 1955.

O'Sullivan, Suzanne. *It's All in Your Head: True Stories of Imaginary Illness.* London: Chatto & Windus, 2015.

Payne, Niravi B. *The Whole Person Fertility Program.* New York: Three Rivers, 1998.

Peck, M. Scott. *People of the Lie: The Hope for Healing Human Evil.* New York: Touchstone, 1998.

Peck, M. Scott. *The Road Less Traveled: A New Psychology of Love, Traditional Values, and Spiritual Growth.* New York: Touchstone, 2012.

Percy, Walker. *Lost in the Cosmos.* New York: Picador, 2000.

Pert, Candace B. *Molecules of Emotion: Why You Feel the Way You Feel.* New York: Simon & Schuster, 1999.

Pirsig, Robert M. *LILA: An Inquiry Into Morals.* New York: Bantam, 1992.

Pirsig, Robert M. *Zen and the Art of Motorcycle Maintenance: An Inquiry Into Values.* New York: Bantam, 1975.

Plasker, Eric. *The 100 Year Lifestyle: Dr. Plasker's Breakthrough Solution for Living Your Best Life Every Day of Your Life!* New York: Adams Media, 2007.

Pollan, Michael. *Food Rules: An Eater's Manual.* New York: Penguin, 2009.

Pollan, Michael. *In Defense of Food: An Eater's Manifesto.* New York: Penguin Press, 2008.

Pollan, Michael. *The Omnivore's Dilemma: A Natural History of Four Meals.* New York: Penguin, 2007.

Pressfield, Steven. *The War of Art: Break Through the Blocks and Win Your Inner Creative Battles.* New York: Warner Books, 2003.

Quindlen, Anna. *A Short Guide to a Happy Life.* New York: Random House, 2020.

Rankin, Lissa. *Mind Over Medicine: Scientific Proof That You Can Heal Yourself.* Carlsbad, CA: Hay House, 2020.

Reynolds, Gretchen. *The First 20 Minutes: Surprising Science Reveals How We Can Exercise Better, Train Smarter, Live Longer.* New York: Avery, 2013.

Roach, Mary. *Gulp: Adventures on the Alimentary Canal.* New York: W. W. Norton, 2014.

Robbins, John. *Healthy at 100: The Scientifically Proven Secrets of the World's Healthiest and Longest-Lived Peoples.* New York: Ballantine, 2007.

Roiphe, Katie. *In Praise of Messy Lives.* New York: The Dial Press, 2012.

Roizen, Michael F. and Mehmet Oz. *You, Staying Young: The Owner's Manual for Extending Your Warranty.* New York: Free Press, 2007.

Rubin, Gretchen. *The Happiness Project.* New York: HarperCollins, 2012.

Rubin, Theodore I. *Compassion and Self-Hate: An Alternative to Despair.* New York: Touchstone, 1998.

Sarno, John E., *The Divided Mind: The Epidemic of Mindbody Disorders.* New York: Harper, 2007.

Sarno, John E. *Healing Back Pain: The Mind-Body Connection.* New York: Balance, 2001.

Sarno, John E. *The Mindbody Prescription: Healing the Body, Healing the Pain.* New York: Warner Books, 1999.

Seneca. *On the Shortness of Life.* New York: Penguin, 2005.

Smith, Julie. *Why Has Nobody Told Me This Before?* New York: Michael Joseph, 2022.

Starrett, Kelly and Glen Cordoza. *Becoming a Supple Leopard: The Ultimate Guide to Resolving Pain, Preventing Injury, and Optimizing Athletic Performance.* Las Vegas: Victory Belt Publishing, 2015.

Starrett, Kelly, Juliet Starrett, and Glen Cordoza. *Deskbound: Standing Up to a Sitting World.* Las Vegas: Victory Belt Publishing, 2016.

Steele, Andrew. *Ageless: The New Science of Getting Older Without Getting Old.* New York: Doubleday, 2021.

Storr, Anthony. *Solitude: A Return to the Self.* New York: Free Press, 2005.

Suzuki, D. T. *An Introduction to Zen Buddhism.* New York: Grove Press, 1964.

Suzuki, David. *The Sacred Balance: Rediscovering Our Place in Nature.* Vancouver: Greystone Books, 2007.

Taubes, Gary. *The Case Against Sugar.* New York: Knopf, 2016.

Taubes, Gary. *Good Calories, Bad Calories: Fats, Carbs, and the Controversial Science of Diet and Health.* New York: Anchor, 2008.

Taubes, Gary. *Why We Get Fat: And What to Do About It.* New York: Anchor, 2011.

Tershakovec, Andrew. *The Mind, The Power That Changed the Planet.* AuthorHouse, 2007.

Thondup, Tulku. *The Healing Power of Mind.* Boulder, CO: Shambhala, 1998.

Tolstoy, Leo. *The Kingdom of God Is Within You.* New York: Cassell Publishing, 1894; Project Gutenberg, 2013. https://www.gutenberg.org/files/43302/43302-h/43302-h.htm.

Topol, Eric. *The Patient Will See You Now: The Future of Medicine Is in Your Hands.* New York: Basic Books, 2016.

Vaillant, George E. *Triumphs of Experience: The Men of the Harvard Grant Study.* Cambridge, MA: Belknap Press, 2015.

Van der Kolk, Bessel. *The Body Keeps the Score: Mind, Brain, and Body in the Transformation of Trauma.* New York: Penguin, 2015.

Volek, Jeff S. and Stephen D. Phinney. *The Art and Science of Low Carbohydrate Living: An Expert Guide to Making the Life-Saving Benefits of Carbohydrate Restriction Sustainable and Enjoyable.* Beyond Obesity, 2011.

Volek, Jeff S. and Stephen D. Phinney. *The Art and Science of Low Carbohydrate Performance.* Beyond Obesity, 2012.

Wahls, Terry and Eve Adamson, *The Wahls Protocol: A Radical New Way to Treat All Chronic Autoimmune Conditions Using Paleo Principles.* New York: Avery, 2014.

Walker, Matthew, *Why We Sleep: Unlocking the Power of Sleep and Dreams.* New York: Scribner, 2017.

Wallace, Meri. *Birth Order Blues: How Parents Can Help their Children Meet the Challenges of their Birth Order.* New York: Holt Paperbacks, 1999.

Ware, Bronnie. *The Top Five Regrets of the Dying: A Life Transformed by the Dearly Departing.* Carlsbad, CA: Hay House, 2012.

Watts, Alan. *Tao: The Watercourse Way.* New York: Pantheon, 1975.

Weil, Andrew. *Spontaneous Healing: How to Discover and Enhance your Body's Natural Ability to Maintain and Heal Itself.* New York: Ballantine, 2000.

Wheelis, Allen. *How People Change.* New York: William Morrow, 1975.

Whitman, Walt. *Leaves of Grass.* United States, 1855; Gutenberg Project 2020. https://gutenberg.org/files/1322/1322-h/1322-h.htm.

Wilber, Ken. *The Integral Vision: A Very Short Introduction to the Revolutionary Integral Approach to Life, God, the Universe, and Everything.* Boulder, CO: Shambhala, 2007.

Wilber, Ken. *The Marriage of Sense and Soul: Integrating Science and Religion.* New York: Harmony, 1999.

Wolpert, Lewis. *How We Live and Why We Die: The Secret Lives of Cells.* New York: W. W. Norton, 2011.

Yalom, Irvin D. *The Gift of Therapy: An Open Letter to a New Generation of Therapists and Their Patients.* New York: Harper, 2017.

Yalom, Irvin D. *Momma and the Meaning of Life, Tales of Psychotherapy.* New York: Harper, 2020.

Yalom, Irvin D. *Staring at the Sun: Overcoming the Terror of Death.* Hoboken, NJ: Jossey-Bass, 2009.

ACKNOWLEDGMENTS

I wish to thank all of the people mentioned in this book, either by name or anonymously, as well as all of the authors of the studies and books I have consulted. The role you played in my life and my education have been profound sources of healing and inspiration.

Others who have supported or contributed to the trajectory of the book and my life (in no intended order) are: Jeffrey Grava, Amrik Dhaliwal, Harvey Langston-Jones, Rachel Kelly, Tania Evans, Kris Carr, Dr. Kirsten Healy, Dr. Oliver Segal, Dr. Cuong Nguyen, Dr. Jason Dolinsky, Kate Pakenham, Weena Pauly-Tarr, NYU Tisch Hospital, Simon Assad, Dana Taylor, Sindhu Porter, Anne and James Andrews, Mark Angelson, Steve Ruggi, Joey Frasier, Dr. Andrew Ferguson, Sophie Ranicar, Peter Manning, Claire Hawkins, Nici Evans, Vanessa Boeye, Ira Fox, Lee Yanqui, Marc Buchner, Sheila Mandell, Vicki Freeman and Mark Meyer, Bobby Kay, William Clark, Marc Lebowitz, Niki and Tim Armacost, Gil Lesko, Meghan Gillespie, and Dr. Lorenzo Masci.

Special thanks to Nikki Costello.

Special thanks to Gail Woodard, Barbara McNichol, Winsome Lewis, and Pam Nordberg.

Special thanks to Jodie Lightfoot.

Special thanks to Graham Fairley.

Special thanks to Marty Keller and John Donovan.

Special thanks to Meri Wallace and Niravi Payne.

Extra special thanks to Jess and Lollie.

And finally, to the great spirit of life that keeps me going and supplied all the energy and inspiration I needed to write it.

ABOUT THE AUTHOR

Ron Kastner embodies a healthy, vibrant, and passionate life after sixty. His unconventional life journey has ranged from being a Woodstock hippie, carpenter, salesman, entrepreneur, investor, advisor, and award-winning theatrical producer.

Becoming a father in his midfifties sparked a transformative shift in Ron's focus for the rest of his life. It centers on health, vitality, longevity, and joy for the purpose of being fully present for his daughters. Along the way, he discovered what is precious about experiencing the universal truths that can be learned from our health and our bodies. Through this book and his blog at RonKastner.com, he shares his practices as well as the wisdom he's gained from this singular yet universal journey focused on physical and spiritual health.

Currently residing in both New York City and London, England, Ron embraces the joys and responsibilities of parenting, writing, and living in his midseventies. Sustained by the love of his two teenage daughters, he maintains a dedicated practice to enhance his longevity and navigate the currents of these precious years well beyond age sixty.

INDEX

A

abdominal breathing, 300
acupuncture treatment, 49–51
aerobic exercise, 58, 175–176
The Aerobics Way (Cooper), 66–67
Africa, experiences in, 96
aging
   calorie restriction, 145
   in horses, 179–180
   misinformation about, 130
   mitigation of processes, 18–19
   movement changes with, 181
   processes of, 16–17
aha moments in daily life, 222–223
alcohol use
   causes of drinking, 92
   negative effects of, 72–74
   relationship effects of, 77–78
   stopping, 75
Anatomy Trains: Myofascial Meridians for Manual and Movement Therapists (Myer), 177
ancient rhythms practice, 215–216
appearance as reflection of health, 263–264
Araujo, Claudio Gil, 181–182
The Art and Science of Low Carbohydrate Living (Volek and Phinney), 148, 150
asanas, 173
attitude, problem-solving and, 211
attractiveness (physique), 65–66

autoimmunity, 24, 33–34
autonomic system (of body)
   functions of, 4
   phases of, 196
   vagus nerve, 86

B

"bad backs", 186
balance
   body fat effects, 184
   components of, 182–183
   expansion of, 186–187
   nature and emotional balance, 189–190
   parasympathetic and sympathetic nervous systems, 196–197
   practicing, 190–191
   sense of inner stability as, 187
   spine and, 184–185, 192
Becoming a Supple Leopard (Starrett), 168, 229
belief
   in beneficial presence, 107
   bodily effects of, 83–85
   physical health and, 113
   role in well-being, 125–126
belly fat, bodily effects of, 184
biological health, factors in, 4
blood tests for health assessment, 231–232
blood type, 147
The Blue Zones, 125–126

body awareness
  as diagnostic tool, 226–227
  in experiencing life, 61–62
  perceived importance of physique, 65–66
  as teacher, 169
  in yoga positions, 186
The Body Keeps the Score (van der Kolk), 62, 178, 284
The Body Never Lies (Miller), 284
bones, muscle and movement support of, 192
BOSU balance trainer, 170
Bowman, Katie, *Move Your DNA*, 168, 206
Brazilian sitting exercise, 230
breathing exercises
  posture and, 285
  for recovery, 208–209
  Wim Hof Method, 113, 209–210
Bucke, Richard, *Cosmic Consciousness*, 260

C

calorie restriction (CR)
  defined, 141
  energy and health effects of, 142–144
Campbell, Joseph
  being who you are, 125
  coming to terms with existence, 106
  divine Transcendent Principle, 108–109
  existence and abilities, source of, 95
  The Masks of God, 213
  Reflections on the Art of Living, 214

cancer, emotional basis of, 91–92
Capital Printing Systems, Inc., 12–14
childhood experiences
  acceptance of, 302–303
  effects in parenting, 240–244, 246–247
circulation for recovery, 206
clarity, grace, wisdom, and serenity, 213–223
clarity, search for, 218–220
Clean (Junger), 22, 25
Clean Gut (Junger), 24
Clean program
  food elimination during, 24
  quiet time during, 25
cloud walk, 191
comfort, evolutionary mismatch symptoms, 256
coming alive, source of, 62
consciousness, development of, 95–96
Cooper, Ken, *The Aerobics Way*, 66–67
Cosmic Consciousness (Bucke), 260
Costello, Nikki, 22, 130–131, 174, 282–283
Crohn's disease, 118
Crowley, Chris, *Younger Next Year*, 18
CURE (Marchant), 86, 122

D

de Grey, Aubrey
  calorie restriction in, 145
  enhancing restorative pathways, 122–123
dead man (land mine) use, 177
"deep health" cleanse program, 23
Deskbound (Starrett), 168

detoxifying
    customized approach to, 24–25
    goals of, 38
    mechanisms of, 28–30
    mental and emotional aspects of, 31–33
    observations during detox, 34–35
    resistance to starting, 34
    restrictions on food for, 25
    serendipitous beginning of, 26
    traditional medical approach to, 47–48
Diamond, Jared, *The World Until Yesterday*, 256–259
"dictatorship of the should" (Karen Horney), 219
diet
    detox elimination diet, 26–27
    importance of, 119
digestion problems, microbiome imbalance, 118
disease
    connections to emotion/inner world, 218
    evolutionary mismatch role in, 255
    self-created emotional component of, 91–92
dis-evolution, 55
Donovan, John, 90
Dyer, Wayne, 114

E

Eastern and Western combination approach, 48–51
The Easy Way to Stop Drinking, 73
eating, role in daily lives, 34
effort and rest cycles, 187
elimination diet, 26–28
emotional biology, 125, 226

emotional detoxing, 25
emotions
    anxiety from, 203–204
    association with disease, 121, 218
    balance for healing, 197
    effects on health, 86
    experiencing vs. thinking of emotion, 96
    role in eating, 144
    triggers of inflammation, 117
    visceral sensations and, 62
emptiness
    broken, 107
    with calorie restriction, 146
    in detoxing, 29–30
engagement with nature, 64–65
enlightenment, 17–18
epigenetics, 269–270
eternal spirit
    alternate name for, 213
    cultivating and harmonizing with, 214
evidence-based approach, 259
evolution
    golden age of human, 114–115
    learning from, 94–95
evolutionary biology, 96
evolutionary mismatch symptoms, 254–256
exercise
    benefits of, 67–68
    copying evolution for, 56–57
    during detoxing, 25, 31
    long and even, 56–57
    short and fast, 57–58
    willpower, motivation, and effort for, 60
    See also movement for health
exertion, 57

Index

F
family, desire for, 97
fascia network
   Anatomy Trains: Myofascial Meridians for Manual and Movement Therapists (Myer), 176
   in movement for health, 176
   in yoga, 173
fasting, body priorities during, 28–30
fat-burning adaptation, 154
fatigue effects in body, 56
fight or flight
   in ancestral lifestyle, 148
   HIIT replication of, 175–176
Food Fix (Hyman), 151
food industry's control over foods, 253
Food Rules (Pollan), 25
Friedman, Howard, *The Longevity Project*, 119
fuel
   in ancestral lifestyle, 148
   eating and modern life, 153
   hunger as DNA-driven instinct, 137
full body movement, 177
functional medicine
   increasing popularity of, 252
   prevention in, 121
   symptom vs. cause treatment in, 118
   treatment approach, 39–41

G
genes, 269–276
gift of life, inner feelings in, 109
glycogen, 147
God, individual nature of, 219–220
Great Guide. *See* eternal spirit

Greenfield, Ben, 168

H
hara hachi bu, 144
have vs. want feelings, 219
Hay, Louise, *Heal Your Body A–Z*, 281
Heal Your Body A–Z (Hay), 281
Healing. *See* eternal spirit
healing
   importance of sleep, 200–201
   inflammation in, 117
   ongoing nature of, 115–116
   rhythms of, 197
   strengthening with, 194
health
   attitude, belief and self-awareness in, 68
   author's definition of, 7–8, 112–113, 122, 228–229
   choices for, 225–235
   diagnostic tool for, 226–229
   as gift at birth, 105–106
   goal of, 118–119
   illness, 277
   inner balance and, 188–189
   meaning of, 35
   practice and training categories for, 124–125
   self-regard effects on, 85
   source of, 4
   taking responsibility for own, 122
health professionals, role in self-care, 233–234
heart problems, 287–297
heart rate variability (HRV), 113, 202
   readiness score from, 230
Help, Thanks, Wow: The Three Essential Prayers (Lamott), 107
Hesse, Herman, *Siddhartha*, 221

high-intensity interval training (HIIT)
   ancestral activity, 175–176
   energy sources for, 147
   for health, 5
Horney, Karen, "dictatorship of the should", 219
How People Change (Wheelis), 246
human evolution
   justice, 257–258
   modern culture mismatch, 254
   positions for rest, 206–207
   treatment of young and old, 258
hunger
   in calorie-restricted diet, 144
   in detoxing, 28–30
   evolutionary mismatch symptoms, 255–256
   ketosis and fat-burning adaptation, 154–155
   role in evolution, 30–31
hunter-gatherer lifestyle
   blueprint for life, 134
   Hadza, 157
Hyman, Mark
   Food Fix, 151, 253
   mind-body connections, 86

I

ikigai (true purpose in life), 9, 125
ill health, 116, 277–300
image (of self)
   false confidence from, 76
   "out front" vs. real, 76–77
immune system
   autoimmunity actions of, 24
   cancer treatment advances in, 252
   evolution of, 137
   functions of, 23
   in healing process, 117
   rhythms of, 196–197
inflammation, 117–119, 148–149
inner life
   guideposts in life, 109
   quality in, 107
inner resources, instinctual rightness, 71
inner stability, 187–188
inspiration
   guidance by, 259
   with Lyme disease, 300
   for writing, 217
instinctual behaviors
   guidance by, 101–102
   guide for health, 81
   parenting, 239–240
   on walking safari, 64
insulin resistance, 149
integrative medical approach
   cause vs. symptom treatment, 118
   increasing popularity of, 252
   prevention in, 121
   role in self-care, 234
intermittent fasting (IF)
   defined, 141
   precedents for, 151–152
interventionist medicine, 42–45, 121
intolerance (foods), 146
irritable bowel disease (IBD), 118
Iyengar, B.K.S.
   Light on Life, 168
   Light on Yoga, 168
   The Iyengar Way (Iyengar), 174

J

Junger, Alejandro
   Clean, 23
   Clean Gut, 22–23

Index

K
Kastner, Ron
  addressing health problems, 202–203
  calorie restriction in practice, 143–144
  cues for healing/recovery, 201
  daily health assessment, 229–230
  daughters, 100–101
  dietary practices of, 141–145
  eating plan, 152
  feelings of failure as father, 101
  genetic story, 270–274
  goals of life, 222
  Golden Rule of parenting, 245
  health goals of, 123–125
  inner guiding force, 106
  morning routine of, 113–114
  recovery methods, 197–199, 204–210
  separation and divorce of, 99
  as single parent, 101–102
  specialty consultants used, 233–234
  typical day of eating, 159–163
  typical day of movement, 169–170
  when bad stuff happens, 277
Keller, Marty, Donovan introduction by, 90
ketosis, 154
kettlebells, 170
Kotelko, Olga, 168

L
Lamott, Anne, *Help, Thanks, Wow: The Three Essential Prayers*, 107
land mine (dead man) use, 177
later life, 9

Leach, Jeffrey, *Rewild*, 157–158
Levitin, Daniel, *Successful Aging*, 130
Lieberman, Daniel, *The Story of the Human Body*, 55, 79, 254–256
Life Spirit. *See* eternal spirit
lifestyle
  buying acceptance, 73–74
  changes to, 8–9, 21
  changes to eating, 25
  cultural and psychic damage of, 256–259
  eating and modern life, 153–154
  gene expression and, 269
  stress on image, 263–267
  three-week detox, 21–22
Light on Life (Iyengar), 168
Light on Yoga (Iyengar), 168
lipoic acid, 156
Lodge, Henry, *Younger Next Year*, 18
longevity
  genes and, 272
  healing role in, 194
  heart rate variability for, 230
  intangible factors in, 69
  predictors of, 119
The Longevity Diet (Longo), 152–153
The Longevity Project (Friedman and Martin), 119
Longo, Valter, *The Longevity Diet*, 152–153
love between spouses, 97–98
loving life, 301–303
low carbohydrate (LC)
  defined, 141
  dietary practices of, 146–151
low-level inflammation, 118
Lyme disease, 277, 297–298

M

Marchant, Jo
  CURE, 86, 122
marriage, 97–98
Martin, Leslie, *The Longevity Project*, 119
The Masks of God (Campbell), 213
Master Linji, *Nothing to Do, Nowhere to Go*, 195
Masters swim team, 175, 193
Maté, Gabor, *The Myth of Normal*, 284
McKeown, Patrick, *The Oxygen Advantage*, 113
meaning in life, support for, 93
metrics, diagnosis, and support, **225–235**
microbiome
  imbalance, 118
  managing gut bacteria, 157–158
micronutrients and supplements, 154–156
Miller, Alice, *The Body Never Lies*, 284
mind-body connections
  back problems, 81–82
  synergistic connections of, 85–86
  tension myositis syndrome (TMS), 82–83
  vagus nerve, 87
modern life
  professional vs. personal needs, 250–251
  shift to prevention in health, 251
modern medicine
  and health, 5–6
  lack of prevention in, 120–121
  message from, 252
  opinions on detoxifying and health, 39–52
  perception of doctors in, 227–228
  shift to preventive and integrative care, 226
mortality moment
  attitude towards exercise shift, 54
  changed beliefs about life, 2–4
  memories of youth, 15–17
  train ride to Jersey, 11–13
Move Your DNA (Bowman), 168, 206
movement for health
  adding movement, 169–172
  aerobic exercise, 175
  becoming sedentary, 66–67
  benefits for bones and joints, 192
  body's need for, 54, 56–60
  comfort vs. movement, 166
  emotional inner life links, 178
  energy sources for, 147
  evolutionary mismatch symptoms, 256
  gym, 174–175
  hard work for connection to body, 166–167
  in human evolution, 165–166
  importance of, 119
  inner awareness with, 178
  instinctual rightness of, 53
  integration into daily life, 169
  lessons in Africa, 62–64
  outdoor and nature time, 172
  as power, 133–134
  rapid results from, 61–62
  rhythms for, 57–58
  supplemental practices, 172–176
  torque and fascia in, 176
  walking and standing, 170–171

Myer, Thomas, *Anatomy Trains: Myofascial Meridians for Manual and Movement Therapists* (Myer), 176
The Myth of Normal (Maté), 284

N

near-term mortality predictor, 181–182
nontraditional healthcare providers, 234
nutrition
  ancestral eating, 140–142
  blood tests for, 156
  body storage of reserves, 147
  diet and health, 138–139
  eating and modern life, 153–154
  eating for recovery, 198–199
  hara hachi bu, 144
  low carbohydrate diet, 149–150
  managing gut bacteria, 157–158
  metabolic balance and healing, 140
  modern diet effects, 138–140
  myths about carbohydrates, 150–151
  supplements and micronutrients, 154–155
  using probiotics, 158–159

O

Oliver, Mary, "Of Power and Time", 93
one-handed bicep pull (TRX strap), 177
The Oxygen Advantage (McKeown), 113
Oz, Mehmet, *You, Staying Young: The Owner's Manual for Extending Your Warranty*, 14–15

P

parenting, 239–247
passion and curiosity, 215
The Patient Will See You Now (Topol), 226
Peck, M. Scott, *The Road Less Traveled*, 97–98, 109
Phinney, Stephen, *The Art and Science of Low Carbohydrate Living*, 148, 150
Pirsig, Robert, *Zen and the Art of Motorcycle Maintenance*, 107, 133
PLAC test, 232
placebo studies, 83–84
Pollan, Michael
  Food Rules, 25
  individual awareness and practice, 253
polo ponies, 179–180
poses (yoga), 173–174, 191
posture, 286. *See also* balance
power, 125
  dynamic and static phases with, 133–134
  experience at yoga retreat, 132
  in health and longevity, 134
  opening channels for, 133
  source and manifestation of, 127–129
Power of the Universe. *See* eternal spirit
pranayama, 209, 285–286
praying/prayer
  for attitude problems, 211
  inspiration and, 107
  in recovery, 106, 210
preventive health practice
  exercise and diet in, 4

preventive health practice (*continued*)
   Junger's theories, 22
   lack of, 52
problems with people, 210
psychological path to healing, 284
psychophysical interactions, 125
psychotherapy
   Donovan support group, 91
   for health, 5, 78
   modern add-on to ancient practices, 217–218
   role in self-care, 234–235
   with separation and divorce, 100
puttering and physical labor, 208

Q
Quality (Pirsig), 107. *See also* power
quality of life, visceral vs. cerebral nature, 110
Quantum Detox, 31

R
rational vs. visceral and emotional faculties, finding your own version of God, 219–220
readiness score, 230
recovery process
   active recovery/restoration, 207
   circulation role in, 206
   conditions for, 211–212
   deep breathing, 208–209
   heart rate variability tool, 205–206
   natural rhythm for, 195
   praying, 210
   puttering and physical labor, 208
   resting positions for, 206–207
   tapering for healing, 194
   time for recovery, 204–205

reduced-symptom living, 118
reflection time in detoxing, 31
relationships
   personal change effects on, 89
   unconventional views and, 78–79
religions, personal experience in, 108–109
renewal, 195–196
repose (in yoga positions), 131
research, 232
resilience
   importance for health, 119–120
   teaching to daughters, 102–103
resting, positions for, 206–207
Rewild (Leach), 157–158
The Road Less Traveled (Peck), 109
Roizen, Michael, *You, Staying Young: The Owner's Manual for Extending Your Warranty*, 14–15

S
Saccharomyces boulardii, 146
sacroiliac joint, 185
Sannyasa, 9
Sarno, John
   mind-body connections, 86
   psychosomatic medicine, 281–284
   tension myositis syndrome, 82
seeking youth, 9
self-care
   defining, 226–229
   for health, 119–121
self-harming habits, source of, 80
self-health fundamentals, 6–7
self-love, subconscious level of, 108
self-parenting, 245
self-realization process, 260–262
self-respect, towards body, 66
senescence, 196

Index

SENS Research Foundation, 122–123
sensory experience
  appreciation of external beauty, 113
  experiencing life on a sensory level, 62
  on walking safari, 63–64
separateness in immune system functions, 33–34
short-term inflammation, 117
sitting-rising test (balance), 181–182
sleep
  benefits of, 198–199
  healing during, 200–201
somatic experiencing (SE), 178
somatic reconnection, 67
spine, effects of curvature, 184
spirituality, 215
standing and walking
  active recovery/restoration, 207–208
  muscles used for, 185–186
  for recovery, 207
Starrett, Kelly
  Becoming a Supple Leopard, 168, 229
  Deskbound, 168
stem cell production, 175
Stick Mobility trainer, 170
"stiff hips", 185
The Story of the Human Body (Lieberman), 55, 79, 254–256
  human evolution, 168
strength training, benefits of, 58–59
Suarez, Michael, 93
success, addictive nature of, 73–74
Successful Aging (Levitin), 130
supplements and micronutrients, 154–156
symbiotic health, 67–68
symptoms
  sources of, 116–117
  treatment of, 118

T

tension myositis syndrome (TMS), 82–83
Thich Nhat Hanh
  Nothing to Do, Nowhere to Go, 195
  walking meditation, 191–192
The Top Five Regrets of the Dying (Ware), 2–3
Topol, Eric, *The Patient Will See You Now*, 226
toxins, effects in body, 29
traditional British/National Health Service approach, 45–46
traditional medical approach, symptom treatment in, 118
TRX belt system, 170, 177
23 and Me testing, 271–272

U

universal force, 133
universal health, bodily senses for, 65
universal power of healing, DNA and freedom, 275
universal self, vs. personal self, 110

V

van der Kolk, Bessel, *The Body Keeps the Score*, 62, 178, 284
vanity, 263–267
visceral bodies/biology
  development of consciousness, 95
  role in well-being, 62
Volek, Jeff, *The Art and Science of Low Carbohydrate Living*, 148

W

Walker, Matthew, *Why We Sleep*, 199
walking meditation, 191–192
walking safari experience, 62–64
Ware, Bronnie, *The Top Five Regrets of the Dying*, 2–3
weight loss
  in calorie-restricted diet, 143–144
  with *Clean* detoxing, 25
well-being
  association with "care", 121
  observations during detox, 31–33
Western medicine. *See* interventionist medicine approach
Wheelis, Allen, *How People Change*, 246
Why We Sleep (Walker), 199
willpower, 79
Wim Hof Method, 113, 209
The World Until Yesterday (Diamond), 256–259
writing for recovery
  free association in, 208
  inner journey from, 216–217
  in summertime, 212

Y

yoga
  awareness of fascia network, 173
  emphasis on spine, 185
  inner body awareness with, 172–173
  Iyengar style, 173
  physical balance practices in, 191
  the poses, 173
  poses for recovery, 207–208

Yoga, The Iyengar Way (Silva and Mehta), 208
You, Staying Young: The Owner's Manual for Extending Your Warranty (Roizen and Oz), 14–15
Younger Next Year (Crowley and Lodge), 18
  biochemistry of exercise, 59–60
  exercise recommendations, 58–59
  experimentation with movement, 168
  medical and evolutionary findings, 54–55

Z

Zen and the Art of Motorcycle Maintenance (Pirsig), 107, 133
Zimmer, Heinrich, 221